GOOD H

*L*OW CALORIE

COOKBOOK

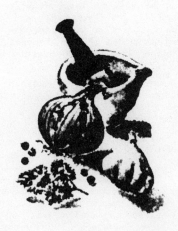

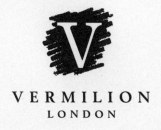

VERMILION
LONDON

Published by Vermilion
an imprint of Ebury Press
Random House
20 Vauxhall Bridge Road
London SW1V 2SA

Second impression 1993

British Library Cataloguing in Publication Data
Good Housekeeping low calorie cookbook: Over 150
recipes to help you watch your weight.
I. Good Housekeeping Institute
641.5

ISBN 0 09 178680 0

Editor: Helen Southall
Nutritionist: Fiona Hunter
Home Economists: Janet Smith, Allyson Birch
Designer: Bob Vickers
Photographer: Ken Field
Additional Photography: James Murphy
Stylist: Maria Jacques
Illustrator: Anne Ormerod

Typeset in Century Old Style by Textype Typesetters, Cambridge
Printed in England by Clays Ltd, St Ives plc

CONTENTS

NOTES

1 The advice and recipes given in this book are intended as a general guide for those who would like to lose weight in a sensible, realistic way. If you are at all worried about any aspect of your health, we strongly recommend that you consult your doctor before following any weight-reduction plan.

2 We have used calories (or kilocalories/kcals) as a measure of energy production throughout this book (see pages 7–8). For those people who prefer to use the standard international unit (the joule) for measuring energy production, one joule (or kilojoule/kj) is equal to 4.2 calories.

USING THE RECIPES

1 Follow either metric or imperial measures for the recipes in this book as they are not interchangeable.

2 All spoon measures are level unless otherwise stated. Sets of measuring spoons are available in both metric and imperial sizes to give accurate measurement of small quantities.

3 When measuring milk, the exact conversion of 568 ml (1 pint) has been used.

4 Size 2 or 3 eggs should be used except where otherwise stated.

5 Raw eggs are used in some recipes. We believe that, at the time of going to press, the proven risk for healthy people using fresh eggs is minimal. However, the elderly, pregnant women, the sick and the very young should avoid eating raw eggs.

*I*NTRODUCTION

*T*HIS is a cookbook about low-calorie, healthy eating; about choosing and using the best ingredients to keep you and your family slim and healthy. Most of us feel the need to shed a few pounds at some point in our lifetime. If you do decide you need to lose weight, it's important to be realistic about your body and the reasons why you want to slim. Nobody should be made to feel that they have to lose weight to conform to fashionable ideas, but it is sensible, for health reasons, to avoid being too fat. So try to forget your fantasies about transforming yourself into a wonderfully glamorous slim new you. Instead, concentrate on developing a generally healthier approach to eating that will keep you fit and well *and* help you to lose weight at the same time.

WHAT IS A HEALTHY DIET?

Fortunately, a diet that will shed unwanted pounds fits in with today's ideas about healthy eating. Over recent years, we've all had the healthy eating principles drummed into us – eat less fat, eat less sugar, eat less salt, eat more fibre. In other words, we should eat less fatty meat, fried foods, butter, margarine, dripping, lard and full-fat dairy products because they are high in fat. Similarly, our consumption of cakes, biscuits and pastries, confectionery, sweetened breakfast cereals, ready-made desserts, fizzy drinks and squashes should be reduced because they all contain lots of sugar. Instead of these fatty and sugary foods we should eat more lean meats, poultry, game, rabbit, offal, fresh fish and low-fat dairy foods such as semi-skimmed milk and low-fat yogurt. Finally, most of us should eat more fibre in the form of fresh fruit and vegetables, unrefined cereals, breakfast cereals, wholemeal bread, pulses, beans, pasta and rice.

By making these alterations to your eating habits and adopting healthier cooking methods (see page 9), you will automatically reduce the number of calories you consume, since the types of food no longer considered healthy are also those that contain most calories.

What about calories?

'Calorie' (with a capital 'C') is a scientific term used by dietitians to measure the amount of energy provided by different amounts and types of food. The same word, 'calorie', but with a small 'C', is used scientifically to describe a much smaller unit of energy that is not practical for everyday use. There are, in fact, 1,000 of these smaller calories in what we usually refer to as a calorie, but which is more correctly expressed as a kilocalorie (kcal).

Energy is produced when food is 'burned up' by the body and is either used up in various ways or stored as body fat, so excess energy produced by excess calories leads to excess weight. In simple terms, the aim of a low-calorie diet is to limit the amount of calories consumed to such a degree that the body has to turn to its fat stores to find the energy it needs.

Obviously, it's particularly important to cut right down on foods which are loaded with calories (usually those high in fat or sugar, as we've just said). When first starting a diet, most people find it helpful to count calories. We all know that a slice of squidgy chocolate gâteau or an ice cream sundae is high in calories, while a lettuce leaf or a dry crispbread is low in calories, but there are things in between! After a while you should be able to recognise high- and low-calorie foods and keep a check on your daily calorie intake without constantly referring to calorie tables. This book is packed with delicious calorie-counted recipes to point you in the right direction. It's useful both for those who have a target weight to reach, and for those who want to follow a sensible, healthy eating plan to maintain their ideal weight.

If you are overweight, you're eating (or have eaten) food containing too many calories for your body's requirements. Different people need different amounts of calories but if the number taken in is about the same as your body uses up, then your weight will stay roughly the same. As we've just said, the key to losing weight is to consume fewer calories than your body needs, so that it starts to use up its stores of fat. It's tempting to try crash diets that cut food intake drastically or restrict your eating to just a couple of foods. If you've tried them already, the chances are that they didn't help you to lose weight permanently, probably because they didn't tackle basic bad eating habits. On any weight-reduction plan you may lose weight rapidly in the first week or so but this is mostly due to water loss rather than fat loss.

So, face up to the fact that there are no miracle cures – the important thing is to change basic eating habits that probably contribute to the problem in the first place.

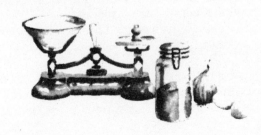

FIRST STEPS TO A SLIMMER, HEALTHIER YOU

Before you begin to worry about counting calories, get into the habit of a healthier way of eating. Train yourself to be aware of what you are eating; think about the ingredients you are buying and the cooking methods you are using. By adopting the following sensible habits it's possible to reduce the calorific value of everyday meals with minimal effort:

- Trim meat of all visible fat.
- Whenever possible, leave skin on vegetables, and eat them raw for maximum goodness.
- Use reduced-fat spreads in place of margarine or butter.
- Reduce your consumption of oil. Replace oils high in saturated fats with those high in polyunsaturated fatty acids, such as corn, soya, sunflower, olive and safflower.
- Don't add sugar to tea, coffee or breakfast cereals. Use artificial sweeteners if you really must.
- Grill or microwave meat and fish instead of frying, or use a heavy-based frying pan brushed very lightly with oil.
- Don't eat snacks between meals.
- Stretch the meat content and improve the nutritive value of casseroles and pies by adding pulses, vegetables or grains.
- Skim surface fat from casseroles. The easiest way to do this is to leave the casserole to cool so the fat rises to the surface and can then be spooned off.
- Use reduced-fat mayonnaise instead of the full-fat version, but remember that even the lower-fat variety should be used in moderation.
- Make dressings with low-fat natural yogurt flavoured with mint, garlic, chilli or herbs, or buy low-calorie dressings.
- Roast meat on a rack in a roasting tin so that the fat can drain off into the tin.
- To make gravies and sauces creamy, add low-fat natural yogurt, fromage frais, reduced-fat cream substitutes or creamy smetana rather than cream. Stir it in at the end of cooking to prevent curdling.
- When a recipe calls for milk, use skimmed or semi-skimmed instead of whole milk.
- To reduce the amount of oil needed, use a heavy-based non-stick pan for things like softening vegetables or cooking omelettes.
- Limit egg consumption to four or five per week.
- Steam vegetables to retain nutrients and flavour. Use vegetable cooking water for sauces, stocks and soups.
- Dry-fry fatty foods, such as bacon and minced meat, in a heavy-based, non-stick pan, cooking them in their own fat. Strain or blot off excess fat with absorbent kitchen paper. Restrict your regular consumption of these foods.

- Remove the skin of poultry before cooking.
- Check labels and avoid any product where fat or sugar comes near the top of the list. Remember that sucrose, glucose, fructose, maltose, dextrose and invert sugar are all forms of sugar.
- Keep a store of calorie-counted meals in your freezer for those days when you don't have the time or the energy to cook.
- Eat baked potatoes topped with cottage cheese, low-fat natural yogurt, fromage frais or baked beans rather than butter or margarine.
- Eat cereals and drink tea and coffee with semi-skimmed or skimmed milk rather than whole milk.
- Limit your consumption of alcohol.
- Drink between six and eight glasses of water each day.
- Always sit down to enjoy your meals, eat slowly and never rush.
- Encourage your family and friends to improve their diets too so that you aren't the odd one out.

HOW DO YOU WEIGH UP?

The chart shown below was produced by the Health Education Authority. It gives the acceptable weight ranges for men and women which carry the least health risk. Draw a horizontal line across the chart for your height

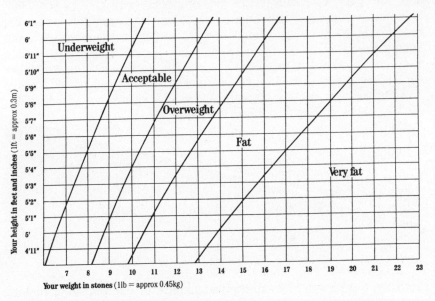

UNDERWEIGHT – Are you eating enough?
ACCEPTABLE – This is the desirable weight range for health.
OVERWEIGHT – Not likely to affect your health but don't get any fatter.
FAT – Your health could suffer if you don't lose weight.
VERY FAT – This is severe and treatment is urgently required.

and a vertical line for your weight; the point where they cross will show you how your weight rates. If you are at the top of the overweight range, or in the fat or very fat range, you should do your best to lose weight.

HOW TO GO ABOUT IT

To lose weight you need to eat less calories than you are eating at present. To calculate your current calorie intake, write down everything you eat and drink for a period of seven days. As you compile the list, try to estimate the weight of the various foods, or if possible, weigh them (for a more accurate calorie count). Having made your list, refer to the chart on pages 155 to 157 to calculate the calorific value of the foods you have eaten. Add up the total calorie intake for the seven days, then divide it by seven to get your average daily calorie intake.

In order to lose weight, dietitians recommend a minimum daily calorie intake of around 1,000 calories for women and 1,500 calories for men. At this level it is usually possible to lose weight gradually and safely. If you are in the 'very fat' category on the chart, this will probably mean reducing your daily intake by about 500 calories. If you are in the 'fat' category, aim to reduce your daily intake by between 200 and 500 calories. (A diet that provides less than 1,000 (1,500) calories is not recommended unless under the supervision of a doctor or dietitian.) Try to keep to your daily allowance for the first couple of weeks. Don't worry about the occasional binge; try to balance your calorie intake throughout the week. If you succeed in sticking to a diet that reduces your calorie intake quite considerably, for some time, you might need to discuss taking a multi-vitamin supplement with your doctor.

Sort out your storecupboard

Having decided to embark on a low-calorie diet, it's sensible to remove all the high-calorie foods out of temptation's way. Re-stocking your storecupboard is a positive way to begin. There are many low- or lower-calorie products on the market that make very good substitutes for everyday foods. Always compare labels; many products which claim to be low-fat or low-calorie are not necessarily what they seem. Read the labels very carefully; many state the calories per 100 g (4 oz) rather than per portion. A portion may well be a lot more than 100 g (4 oz).

The following suggestions are a good start:

- Replace high-sugar preserves with high-fruit, low-sugar jams and spreads (keep in the refrigerator once opened).
- Discard all shop-bought gooey cakes and biscuits. Replace with plain biscuits, for emergencies only.
- Replace breakfast cereals and muesli containing sugar with high-fibre, no-sugar varieties.

- Replace canned fish in oil with fish in brine or water.
- Replace ordinary baked beans with low-sugar, low-salt varieties.
- Replace peanut butter with a no-added-salt-or-sugar brand. Eat in small quantities; it is very high in calories.
- Buy fruits canned in natural unsweetened fruit juice rather than syrup.
- Buy wholemeal bread in preference to white; it's more filling.
- Buy good quality, tasty, high-fibre bread and learn to enjoy it without butter or margarine.
- Buy dried skimmed milk powder in preference to dried whole milk.
- Buy fat-reduced drinking chocolate in preference to the full-fat variety.
- Buy canned tomatoes and tomato purée. They are excellent for making quick, low-calorie pasta sauces or adding to casseroles, or as a basis for quick soups.
- Buy tomato ketchup made without added sugar.

Re-stock your fridge

After sorting out your storecupboard, it's a good idea to re-stock your fridge too. Dairy products are very high in calories because they contain a lot of fat (of the undesirable saturated kind). Replace them wherever possible with lower-fat alternatives. In some cases you will hardly notice the difference: semi-skimmed milk tastes the same as full-fat milk but has half the fat, and fat means calories! Low-fat spreads can be used successfully for softening vegetables, on toast and for baking in some recipes. So take action now! Implement the suggestions below to make your fridge a low-calorie zone.

- Replace full-fat milk with semi-skimmed milk or skimmed milk.
- Replace full-fat hard cheese with reduced-fat cheeses or medium-fat hard cheese such as Edam, or soft cheese like Camembert.
- Replace full-fat cream cheese with reduced-fat cream cheese or low-fat yogurt, fromage frais, quark or smetana.
- Replace full-fat mayonnaise with a fat-reduced brand.
- Replace high-sugar fizzy drinks with low-calorie versions or, better still, mineral water.
- Replace butter with fat-reduced butter or fat-reduced spread.
- Buy lots of fresh fruit for a low-calorie dessert or to nibble between meals.
- Buy lots of fresh vegetables to add low-calorie bulk and nutrients to all meals.
- Keep a bottle of mineral or soda water chilled, ready to dilute white wine and fruit juices.
- Buy chicken and white fish in preference to red meats.
- Buy low-calorie mixers and drinks.
- Replace full-fat, sweetened fruit yogurts with low-fat, low-sugar, real fruit varieties.

Know your weaknesses

At certain times many of us eat out of habit rather than hunger. Try to identify and avoid places, people, moods, times and situations that cause you to eat more than you intend. For instance, if you find that you pick on peanuts and crisp snacks in wine bars and pubs, try to entertain more at home (with the help of our delicious menus on pages 127–154) where you know you have more control over the food, or go to a pub where crisps and peanuts aren't for sale. Teach yourself not to pick while preparing meals, and don't automatically reach for the biscuit tin when you make a cup of tea or coffee.

Never go shopping on an empty stomach; write a list and stick to it! Don't buy crisps or biscuits for your family if you know that you won't be able to resist them. Avoid walking home from work via the sweet shop if you know you are always tired and in need of a 'treat' at that time of the day. If you tend to pick at biscuits, cakes or bread and cheese while watching television or when you are bored, keep busy! Avoid friends who encourage overeating and drinking until you are confident with your diet, or better still, encourage them to join you in your weight-reduction plan!

The importance of breakfast

Get the day off to a good start with a filling, well-balanced breakfast. It really is worth making time for; you are less likely to pick at mid-morning snacks if you have eaten properly at breakfast time. We haven't included breakfast recipes in this book because the simplest, quickest things we all know are best.

A high-fibre (unsweetened) cereal with semi-skimmed milk is 260 kcals. A poached egg on toast with low-fat spread is 175 kcals. A bacon sandwich made with lean grilled bacon and tomato is about 260 kcals. Coffee and tea without sugar or milk is virtually calorie-free. The rules of healthy eating apply: avoid frying – poach, boil or scramble eggs (with low-fat spread in a non-stick pan); grill lean bacon, or dry-fry in a non-stick frying pan and blot off excess fat; grilled low-fat sausages should be reserved for an occasional treat. Choose unsweetened breakfast cereals and serve with skimmed or semi-skimmed milk, or porridge with fruit and a little honey or salt to taste. Spread toast thinly with low-fat spread and low-sugar marmalade, jam or yeast extract. Orange juice is about 50 kcals a serving; drink it diluted half and half with sparkling mineral water. In the summer, a fresh fruit salad made with various fruits in season, moistened with apple or orange juice, and served with low-fat natural yogurt makes a refreshing start to the day. Finally, don't neglect the all-time dieters' favourite – the grapefruit. One serving is only 15 kcals.

Alcohol

While on a diet, it's advisable to reduce your consumption of alcohol. It contains no nutrients and is an easy way of piling on the calories with little effort. It's also an appetite stimulant; a few glasses can crush even the strongest will-power.

Most people don't realise just how many calories alcoholic drinks contain. A glass of sweet white wine is 105 kcals, while spirits, such as gin and vodka, are 60 kcals per measure. Just three gin and tonics would use up almost one third of the day's calorie allowance! There's no need to give up alcohol altogether, but try to restrict your intake to one or two units per week. (A unit is one glass of wine, one measure of spirit or half a pint of lager.) Never let anyone fill up your glass until it is completely empty or you'll lose track of how much you've had. To make a glass of wine go further, try diluting it with sparkling mineral water or soda water and lots of ice to make a refreshing spritzer.

When diluting spirits with mixers, use low-calorie tonic and put that into the glass before adding the spirit. Don't mix it; you will find that the drink has a stronger alcoholic punch than if mixed the conventional way because the smell of the spirit hits you as you lift the glass to drink. You can almost convince yourself that it's a double! Don't make the mistake of opting for fruit juice instead of alcohol – 300 ml (½ pint) orange juice is almost twice as calorific as a measure of spirit. Low-alcohol wines are half the calories or less of their alcoholic counterparts but tend to be sweet and fizzy. Alcohol-free or low-alcohol lagers are a better bet as they are about half the calories of the real thing and taste quite pleasant.

Eating out

Being on a diet doesn't mean that eating out is impossible. Of course it helps if you are a regular at a favourite restaurant where you can explain to the staff that you must avoid fatty and sugary foods. (Imply medical reasons – it gets better co-operation!) Otherwise, you should stick to those foods on the menu that you know are included in your diet. Beware of calorie-laden starters, such as pâté and avocado. Choose melon (only 15 kcals per serving), smoked salmon or consommé instead. Specify that you want your fish grilled and served without buttery sauce, or choose the plainest poultry or meat dish on the menu. Avoid anything fried. Vegetarian dishes are not automatically low in calories; watch out for nuts and cheese. Ask for vegetables without butter and salad with dressing served separately. If pasta is on the menu, choose a tomato-based sauce in preference to a creamy sauce. Watch out for the waiter who lavishes Parmesan cheese on top – it adds an extra 60 kcals per 15 ml (1 tbsp)! For pudding, choose fresh fruit or fruit salad, but check that the latter isn't soaking in sugary syrup. Cheese and biscuits can have as many calories as a pudding – fruit is far better.

Having said all this, if you're going out for a meal you might as well enjoy it. Try to plan ahead 'calorie wise' for special occasions, business lunches and birthdays. Don't worry about consuming a few calories too many during one meal, simply compensate by having a few really 'good' days afterwards.

Exercise

Remember that regular exercise is important, too. It burns up some calories (though not as many as we are sometimes led to believe), but more importantly it helps you get fit, tones up flabby muscles and generally promotes a feeling of well-being. If your life is not ordered enough to fit in regular classes, try walking or cycling to work instead of taking the bus, or go swimming a couple of times a week. Don't use a lift or escalator when you could use the stairs. In other words – keep on the move as much as you can!

Checking your progress

On any weight-reduction plan, you may lose weight rapidly in the first week or so, but that's mostly due to loss of body water rather than fat. After the first week or two on a sensible diet you should feel pleased with yourself if you're losing a steady ½–1 kg (1–2 lb) a week. Resist the temptation to weigh yourself each time you pass the scales. Your body weight will fluctuate from day to day. To check any real weight loss, weigh yourself weekly, preferably in the morning before breakfast. Always wear clothes of a similar kind – jeans and a thick jumper add more pounds than a thin skirt and T-shirt. Even without scales, it's easy to check your progress – after a couple of weeks you should notice that your clothes are looser.

STAYING SLIM

Having reached your ideal weight, you will want to maintain it at that level. It should be possible to increase your daily intake of calories without putting on weight. It will be a case of trial and error. If you eat too much you will soon know because your weight will go up and your clothes will start to feel tight again! Remember that the recipes in this book are delicious enough to eat at any time, not just when on a strict diet. By referring to them for your everyday meals it will be easy to stay healthy, well fed *and* slim!

SATISFYING SOUPS

HOME-MADE soups are delicious to eat and satisfying to make. While on a calorie-controlled diet, they make a filling, low-calorie meal for lunch or supper, or, when served in smaller quantities, they can be a welcoming start to a simple meal.

Try to make soup with home-made stock; it has a much more intense flavour and is lower in salt than stock made from cubes. Make up a large batch, leave to cool, then remove the layer of fat from the top before storing. Stock can be kept in the refrigerator for up to one week, but it should be boiled every 1–2 days. It also freezes well – reduce it to a small concentrated quantity and freeze in ice cube trays. Dilute with water when required.

Traditional accompaniments to soup can be high in calories. Try some new alternatives:

- Instead of frying bread croûtons, make them from toasted slices of bread, cut into dice.
- Swirl yogurt on top of soup instead of cream.
- Give puréed chilled soups extra texture by garnishing with a julienne of carrot or spring onion, or with thin slices of cucumber, courgette, radish or apple.
- Grated hard cheese adds protein and flavour. Use a fat-reduced variety to lower the calories.
- Beware of munching your way through lots of bread with your soup; even without butter, it adds an extra 65 kcals per slice to your meal.

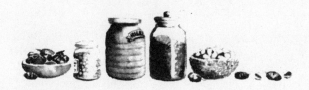

SPICED LENTIL AND CARROT SOUP

This is a warming substantial soup for cold, wintry days. Serve for a family supper.

Serves 4

98 kcals per serving

15 ml (1 tbsp) vegetable oil
200 g (7 oz) carrots, peeled and
    grated
1 medium onion, skinned and finely
    sliced

10 whole green cardamoms
50 g (2 oz) split red lentils
1.2 litres (2 pints) chicken stock
salt and freshly ground pepper
parsley sprigs, to garnish

1 Heat the oil in a heavy-based saucepan, add the carrots and onion and cook gently for 4–5 minutes.
2 Meanwhile, split each cardamom and remove the black seeds. Crush the seeds in a pestle and mortar, or use the end of a rolling pin on a wooden board.
3 Add the crushed cardamom seeds to the vegetables with the lentils. Cook, stirring, for a further 1–2 minutes.
4 Add the chicken stock and bring to the boil. Lower the heat, cover and simmer gently for about 20 minutes or until the lentils are just tender. Season to taste with salt and pepper. Serve hot, garnished with parsley sprigs.

CREAMY LETTUCE SOUP

Use some of the dark green leaves from the outside of the lettuce to give the soup a good colour.

Serves 4

145 kcals per serving

1 medium cos lettuce, weighing about
    450 g (1 lb)
1 medium onion, skinned
1 small potato, peeled

25 g (1 oz) low-fat spread
300 ml (½ pint) vegetable stock
450 ml (¾ pint) semi-skimmed milk
salt and freshly ground pepper

1 Wash the lettuce thoroughly, then chop roughly. Finely chop the onion and potato. For speed, the vegetables can all be whirled together in a blender or food processor for a few seconds.

2 Melt the low-fat spread in a medium saucepan and sauté the vegetables for 4–5 minutes or until well coated and beginning to soften. Pour on the stock and milk. Bring to the boil, cover and simmer gently for 15–20 minutes or until all the vegetables are tender.

3 Leave the soup to cool slightly, then purée in a blender or food processor, or rub through a sieve. Reheat the soup gently and season with salt and pepper to taste before serving.

WATERCRESS SOUP

Try serving this delicately flavoured soup with a swirl of Greek yogurt over the top of each bowl, adding only a few calories to each serving.

Serves 4

95 kcals per serving

15 ml (1 tbsp) vegetable oil
1 small onion, skinned and chopped
1 bunch of watercress, trimmed and
   coarsely chopped
20 g (¾ oz) plain flour
300 ml (½ pint) vegetable stock

300 ml (½ pint) semi-skimmed milk
1.25 ml (¼ tsp) grated nutmeg
salt and freshly ground pepper
watercress sprigs and paprika, to
   garnish

1 Heat the oil in a medium heavy-based saucepan. Add the onion and watercress and cook over a low heat for 3–5 minutes, stirring occasionally, until the onion is soft but not brown.

2 Add the flour and cook for 1 minute, then gradually stir in the stock, milk and nutmeg. Bring to the boil, stirring. Season with salt and pepper to taste, lower the heat, cover, and simmer for about 15 minutes or until thickened and smooth.

3 Remove from the heat and leave to cool slightly, then purée in a blender or food processor until smooth. Return the soup to the saucepan. Reheat gently and serve in warmed individual bowls garnished with watercress sprigs and a sprinkling of paprika.

CREAM OF PARSLEY SOUP

Parsley is very rich in a number of essential minerals, including calcium, iron and potassium.

Serves 4

113 kcals per serving

25 g (1 oz) low-fat spread
225 g (8 oz) floury potatoes, peeled and thinly sliced
1 onion, skinned and finely sliced
100 g (4 oz) chopped fresh parsley

300 ml (½ pint) vegetable stock
300 ml (½ pint) semi-skimmed milk
salt and freshly ground pepper
low-fat natural yogurt, to garnish

1   Melt the low-fat spread in a medium saucepan and add the potatoes, onion and parsley. Cook over a medium heat for 5–10 minutes or until the potatoes begin to soften, stirring constantly.
2   Add the stock, milk and salt and pepper to taste, and simmer for 30 minutes. Leave the soup to cool slightly, then purée in a blender or food processor until very smooth. Reheat the soup gently and serve in warmed individual bowls with a swirl of yogurt on top.

BROCCOLI AND ORANGE SOUP

This unusual combination of flavours makes a very refreshing soup, ideal for serving at a summer lunch.

Serves 4

93 kcals per serving

350 g (12 oz) broccoli, divided into stalks and small florets
900 ml (1½ pints) chicken stock
25 g (1 oz) low-fat spread
1 onion, skinned and chopped

25 g (1 oz) plain flour
150 ml (¼ pint) semi-skimmed milk
rind and juice of 1 large orange, with rind cut into fine strips
salt and freshly ground pepper

1 Peel the broccoli stalks if thick and roughly chop. Set aside with half the broccoli florets.

2 Bring the stock to the boil in a medium saucepan. Add the remaining florets and simmer for 3 minutes. Strain the broccoli florets, reserving the stock, and set aside.

3 Melt the low-fat spread in a heavy-based saucepan, add the onion and cook gently for 5 minutes. Add the flour and cook, stirring, for 1 minute.

4 Gradually add the stock, stirring until thickened and smooth. Add the uncooked broccoli stalks and florets. Simmer, covered, for 25 minutes.

5 Leave the soup to cool slightly, then purée in a blender or food processor until smooth. Return to the pan with the milk, 2.5 ml ($\frac{1}{2}$ tsp) of the orange rind, the orange juice and salt and pepper to taste. Reheat gently.

6 Before serving, add the cooked broccoli florets to the soup and reheat. Serve in warmed bowls, sprinkled with the remaining orange rind.

WHITE BEAN SOUP

Pecorino is a delicious strong-flavoured Italian cheese available from delicatessens and Italian food shops. Serve this soup as a supper dish.

Serves 4

255 kcals per serving

15 ml (1 tbsp) vegetable oil
1 medium onion, skinned and finely chopped
1 garlic clove, skinned and crushed
10 ml (2 tsp) chopped fresh rosemary or 2.5 ml ($\frac{1}{2}$ tsp) dried
425 g (15 oz) can haricot beans, drained and rinsed

1.2 litres (2 pints) vegetable stock
salt and freshly ground pepper
100 g (4 oz) Pecorino or Lancashire cheese, thinly sliced
toasted wholemeal bread croûtons and sprigs of fresh rosemary, to garnish

1 Heat the oil in a large heavy-based saucepan and sauté the onion with the garlic and rosemary for 1–2 minutes. Add the beans, stock and salt and pepper to taste. Bring to the boil, cover and simmer for 10 minutes.

2 Leave the soup to cool slightly, then purée half in a blender or food processor and return to the pan. Bring back to the boil, stirring all the time. Adjust the seasoning.

3 Serve the soup with wafers of Pecorino or Lancashire cheese, wholemeal bread croûtons and fresh rosemary.

MUSSEL CHOWDER

If fresh mussels are not available, use 175 g (6 oz) frozen shelled mussels, thawed. Add to the soup as directed for the fresh mussels, and use fish stock in place of the cooking liquid.

Serves 4

145 kcals per serving

1.2 litres (2 pints) fresh mussels, well scrubbed
15 ml (1 tbsp) vegetable oil
1 small green pepper, cored, seeded and finely chopped
1 onion, skinned and finely chopped
3 celery sticks, trimmed and finely chopped

1 garlic clove, skinned and chopped
400 g (14 oz) can chopped tomatoes
1 bay leaf
15 ml (1 tbsp) chopped fresh thyme or 7.5 ml (1½ tsp) dried
salt and freshly ground pepper
chopped fresh parsley and the finely pared rind of 1 lemon, to garnish

1 Place the mussels in a large saucepan and add 300 ml (½ pint) water. Cover and bring to the boil. Cook gently for a few minutes, until the mussel shells have opened.

2 Meanwhile, heat the oil in a non-stick saucepan. Add the green pepper, onion, celery and garlic and cook gently for about 5 minutes or until soft.

3 Drain the mussels, reserving the liquid, and discarding any unopened ones. Shell the mussels, reserving four in their shells for garnish.

4 Make the reserved cooking liquid up to 450 ml (¾ pint) with cold water, if necessary, and add to the vegetables with the tomatoes and their juice, the bay leaf, thyme and salt and pepper to taste. Bring to the boil, cover and simmer for 25 minutes.

5 Add the shelled mussels to the soup and cook for a further 5 minutes. Remove the bay leaf and adjust the seasoning. Ladle the soup into warmed serving bowls, add a mussel in its shell to each bowl and garnish with parsley and lemon rind.

SPRING PRAWN SOUP

Prawns are a low-fat source of protein, as is yogurt. Serve this chilled soup as a dinner-party starter.

Serves 4

181 kcals per serving

275 g (10 oz) cooked prawns, peeled with shells reserved
2 spring onions, chopped
1 small bunch of parsley stalks
1 bay leaf
1 strip of thinly pared lemon rind
300 ml (½ pint) dry white wine

salt and freshly ground pepper
20 g (¾ oz) low-fat spread
20 g (¾ oz) plain flour
150 ml (5 fl oz) low-fat natural yogurt
lemon slices and fresh dill sprigs, to garnish

1 Place the prawn shells in a saucepan with the spring onions, parsley stalks, bay leaf, lemon rind and 600 ml (1 pint) water. Bring to the boil, lower the heat, cover and simmer gently for 25 minutes.

2 Pour the prawn stock through a fine sieve and discard the shells and flavourings. Mix with the white wine, season with salt and pepper to taste and reserve.

3 Melt the low-fat spread in a heavy-based pan, stir in the flour and cook for 1 minute. Gradually stir in the reserved stock and bring to the boil. Lower the heat, add two-thirds of the prawns and simmer gently for about 5 minutes. Leave to cool slightly, then purée in a blender or food processor until smooth. Set aside to cool, then stir in the yogurt. Chill for 3–4 hours.

4 Stir the remaining prawns into the soup. Serve garnished with lemon slices and sprigs of dill.

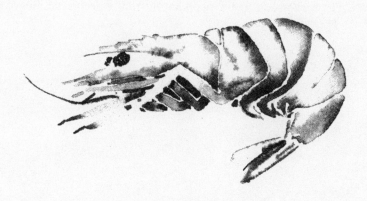

*C*ARIBBEAN SPINACH AND CRAB SOUP

This soup is spicily hot and very tasty. Serve it as an unusual starter for a dinner party, then follow with a Caribbean-style main course of grilled chicken. Bananas simmered in orange juice with a pinch of ground all-spice would complete the West Indian theme of the meal.

Serves 6

111 kcals per serving

450 g (1 lb) fresh spinach
25 g (1 oz) low-fat spread
4 spring onions, trimmed and chopped
2 large garlic cloves, skinned and crushed
30 ml (2 tbsp) plain flour
30 ml (2 tbsp) desiccated coconut

5 ml (1 tsp) cayenne
1.2 litres (2 pints) fish or vegetable stock
salt and freshly ground pepper
170 g (6 oz) can white crab meat in brine
few drops of Tabasco sauce (optional)

1 Trim and wash the spinach and chop the leaves roughly, discarding any thick or tough stalks.
2 Melt the low-fat spread in a large heavy-based saucepan, add the onions and garlic and fry gently for 5 minutes or until soft but not coloured.
3 Add the spinach and cook gently for 2–3 minutes, then stir in the flour, coconut and cayenne. Pour in the stock and bring to the boil, stirring, then add salt and pepper to taste. Lower the heat, cover and simmer for 20 minutes, stirring occasionally.
4 Add the crab meat and brine to the soup and heat through for at least 5 minutes, stirring gently. Taste and adjust the seasoning and add a dash of Tabasco if a more pronounced 'peppery' flavour is preferred. Serve hot.

CHICKEN AND PRAWN GUMBO

Gumbo is the American term for okra, which is sometimes also known as 'ladies' fingers'. Its slightly gelatinous quality when cooked is used to thicken soups and stews.

Serves 8 or 10

273 or 219 kcals per serving

50 g (2 oz) streaky bacon, rinded and chopped
2 garlic cloves, skinned and finely chopped
1 large onion, skinned and finely chopped
15 ml (1 tbsp) plain flour
2 tomatoes, skinned and chopped
1 green pepper, cored, seeded and finely sliced
1 bay leaf
1.2 litres (2 pints) chicken stock

175 g (6 oz) long grain rice
225 g (8 oz) okra
450 g (1 lb) cooked chicken meat, skinned and diced
450 g (1 lb) peeled cooked prawns, thawed if frozen
few drops of Tabasco sauce
few drops of Worcestershire sauce
salt and freshly ground pepper
whole cooked crayfish, to garnish (optional)

1 In a large heavy-based saucepan, cook the bacon gently in its own fat for 2–3 minutes or until transparent. Add the garlic and onion and fry gently for about 7 minutes or until golden.
2 Sprinkle in the flour. Stir well, cook for 1–2 minutes, then remove from the heat.
3 Add the tomatoes and green pepper with the bay leaf and stock. Stir well, return to the heat and bring to the boil. Cover and simmer for 20 minutes. Add the rice and boil for a further 10 minutes.
4 Trim the okra and slice evenly into rings. Add to the gumbo with the chicken and prawns, then add the Tabasco and Worcestershire sauces with salt and pepper to taste.
5 Simmer for 10 minutes or until heated through. Ladle the gumbo into a warmed soup tureen and serve hot, garnishing each portion with a whole crayfish, if available.

CURRIED CHICKEN SOUP

Garam masala is a combination of Indian spices, and is available at most supermarkets and specialist shops.

Serves 4

165 kcals per serving

1 onion, skinned and chopped
100 g (4 oz) split red lentils
5 ml (1 tsp) ground turmeric
5 ml (1 tsp) garam masala
2.5 ml (½ tsp) chilli powder, or to taste
900 ml (1½ pints) chicken stock

225 g (8 oz) cooked chicken meat,
  skinned and coarsely chopped
salt and freshly ground pepper
low-fat natural yogurt, fresh parsley
  sprigs and paprika, to garnish

1 Put the onion, lentils, spices, stock and half the chicken into a medium saucepan. Bring to the boil, lower the heat, cover and simmer for 20 minutes. Leave to cool slightly, then purée in a blender or food processor.
2 Return the mixture to the pan and add the remaining chicken. Heat gently, then simmer for a further 10 minutes. Season with salt and pepper to taste and serve garnished with yogurt, parsley and paprika.

COCK-A-LEEKIE SOUP

A substantial soup to serve with wholemeal bread for a hearty lunch or supper dish.

Serves 6

91 kcals per serving

15 ml (1 tbsp) vegetable oil
275–350 g (10–12 oz) chicken (1
  large or 2 small chicken portions)
350 g (12 oz) leeks, trimmed
1.2 litres (2 pints) chicken stock

1 bouquet garni
salt and freshly ground pepper
6 prunes, stoned
parsley sprigs, to garnish

1 Heat the oil in a large heavy-based saucepan and fry the chicken quickly until golden on all sides.

2 Cut the white part of each leek lengthways into four and chop into 2.5 cm (1 inch) pieces. (Reserve the green parts.) Add the white parts to the pan and fry for 5 minutes or until soft.

3 Add the stock, bouquet garni and salt and pepper to taste. Bring to the boil and simmer for 30 minutes or until the chicken is tender.

4 Shred the reserved green parts of the leeks, then add to the pan with the prunes. Simmer for a further 30 minutes.

5 To serve, remove the chicken, then cut the meat into large pieces, discarding the skin and bones. Place the meat in a warmed soup tureen. Taste and adjust the seasoning of the soup, remove the bouquet garni, and pour over the chicken. Serve hot, garnished with parsley sprigs.

*C*HILLED SPRING ONION SOUP

Make double the quantity of this simple soup and freeze the leftovers for up to 3–4 months.

Serves 4

109 kcals per serving

15 spring onions
40 g (1½ oz) low-fat spread
2 potatoes, peeled and sliced
3 celery sticks, trimmed and chopped

salt and freshly ground pepper
150 ml (5 fl oz) low-fat natural yogurt
extra yogurt, to garnish

1 Trim the green tops from the spring onions and reserve. Trim off the root ends, then roughly chop the onion bulbs. Melt the low-fat spread in a medium heavy-based saucepan and add the potatoes, celery and chopped spring onion bulbs. Cook, stirring, for about 1 minute, then add 600 ml (1 pint) cold water. Bring to the boil, stir, cover and simmer for 15–20 minutes or until the vegetables are soft.

2 Leave the soup to cool slightly, then purée in a blender or food processor until smooth. Season with salt and pepper to taste and leave to cool for about 4 hours.

3 Whisk the yogurt into the cooled soup and add a little water to thin the soup, if necessary. Chill for 1 hour. Serve chilled, garnished with chopped spring onion tops and extra yogurt.

*M*ARBLED ICED BORSHCH

If you prefer a smooth borshch, purée in a blender or food processor after cooking in step 4.

Serves 6

95 kcals per serving

225 g (8 oz) chuck steak, trimmed of all fat
1 carrot, scrubbed and sliced
1 onion, skinned and stuck with a few cloves
2 celery sticks, trimmed and chopped
1 bouquet garni
salt and freshly ground pepper
350 g (12 oz) raw beetroot

225 g (8 oz) ripe tomatoes, skinned and roughly chopped
30 ml (2 tbsp) tomato purée
15 ml (1 tbsp) red wine vinegar
1 bay leaf
5 ml (1 tsp) sugar, or to taste
150 ml (5 fl oz) low-fat natural yogurt, to serve

1   Put the beef in a large saucepan with the carrot, onion and celery. Pour in 1.2 litres (2 pints) water and bring to the boil. Skim off any scum and add the bouquet garni and salt and pepper to taste. Lower the heat, cover and simmer for 1 hour or until the meat is just becoming tender.
2   Meanwhile, peel the beetroot and cut into thin, matchstick strips with a very sharp knife.
3   Remove the beef from the pan and slice into thin matchstick strips, as with the beetroot. Remove the vegetables and bouquet garni with a slotted spoon and discard.
4   Return the beef to the pan and add the beetroot, tomatoes, tomato purée, wine vinegar and bay leaf. Simmer for a further 50 minutes to 1 hour or until the beef and beetroot are really tender. Discard the bay leaf, then adjust the seasoning, adding sugar to taste. Transfer the soup to a bowl and chill for 3–4 hours or overnight.
5   To serve the borshch, pour it into a soup tureen or individual serving bowls, then carefully swirl in the yogurt to create a marbled pattern.

SLIMLINE SUPPERS AND LUNCHES

SUPPERTIME is the downfall of many dieters. For workers returning home hungry and in a rush to eat something quick, or non-workers tired because it's the end of the day, calorie counting is the last thing on the mind. Bread, cheese and biscuits are instantly gratifying and available, but high in calories! This chapter contains lots of tempting recipes suitable for both lunch and supper that are low in calories. Many are quick and easy to make. If you know that the evening is your 'picking' time, try to plan ahead. Cook meals in batches and freeze for use later in the week.

If you are working, a home-made lunch is difficult. Packed lunches are an answer, but for most of us they are impractical. If you rely on a canteen or sandwich bar, choose low-calorie options, like a baked potato (without butter) topped with cottage cheese or baked beans, or a wholemeal sandwich filled with smoked salmon and cucumber, tuna fish or chicken with salad, lean ham and tomato. Salads, the traditional dieters' lunch, are not automatically low in calories. Many are drenched in high-calorie dressing and should be avoided unless the dressing is served separately or they are of the pre-packed, calorie-counted variety. At weekends, lunch shouldn't be a problem – just look through the recipes in this chapter and you'll be spoilt for choice.

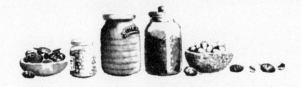

STEAMED MUSSELS IN PEPPER BROTH

Always buy more mussels than you need as a few will be discarded before and after cooking. Allow about 350 g (12 oz) per person for a starter and 450 g (1 lb) per person for a main course.

Serves 6

126 kcals per serving

4 kg (4½ lb) fresh mussels
salt and freshly ground pepper
a little oatmeal
15 ml (1 tbsp) olive oil
1 medium onion, skinned and finely
  chopped

2 large red peppers, cored, seeded
  and finely chopped
2 bay leaves
1 garlic clove, skinned and crushed
450 g (1 lb) tomatoes, chopped
45 ml (3 tbsp) chopped fresh dill

1 Discard any cracked mussels and any that remain open when tapped sharply on the shell. Scrub the mussels, pull off the coarse threads (beards) from the sides of the shells and soak in cold water, with a little salt and oatmeal added, for at least 30 minutes or overnight.
2 Heat the oil in a medium, heavy-based saucepan. Add the onion, most of the red pepper (reserving some for garnish), 1 bay leaf and the garlic. Sauté for about 5 minutes or until beginning to soften. Add the tomatoes and cook, stirring, for 1–2 minutes before adding 600 ml (1 pint) water. Bring to the boil, cover and simmer for about 15 minutes. Leave the mixture to cool slightly, then purée in a blender or food processor. Sieve into a clean saucepan and add salt and pepper to taste.
3 Drain and rinse the mussels and place in a large saucepan. Add 150 ml (¼ pint) water and the remaining bay leaf. Cover the pan tightly and place over a high heat. Steam the mussels, shaking the pan occasionally, for 3–5 minutes. After cooking, discard any mussels that have not opened.
4 Strain the cooking liquid from the mussels into the pepper broth. Stir in the chopped dill and bring to the boil. Adjust the seasoning. Divide the mussels among six individual serving bowls and pour over the pepper broth. Garnish with the reserved diced red pepper.

*T*UNA AND DILL FISH CAKES

These are a healthy alternative to traditional fish cakes. Cooked in the oven, they are high in protein but low in fat.

Serves 4

306 kcals per serving

225 g (8 oz) potatoes, scrubbed
15 g (½ oz) low-fat spread
30 ml (2 tbsp) low-fat natural yogurt
two 200 g (7 oz) cans tuna in brine, drained and flaked
40 ml (2½ tbsp) chopped fresh dill or 15 ml (1 tbsp) dried
15 ml (1 tbsp) grated onion
grated rind of 1 lemon
freshly ground pepper
15 ml (1 tbsp) plain flour
2 egg whites, beaten
75 g (3 oz) dried breadcrumbs or rolled oats
45 ml (3 tbsp) reduced-fat mayonnaise
lemon wedges and fresh dill, to garnish

1 Cook the potatoes in boiling water for 20 minutes or until tender. Drain and peel, then add the low-fat spread and 15 ml (1 tbsp) of the yogurt. Mash until smooth, then turn into a mixing bowl and leave to cool.
2 Add the tuna, 25 ml (1½ tbsp) fresh dill or 10 ml (2 tsp) dried dill, the onion, lemon rind and pepper to taste to the potato. Mix well, cover and chill for about 15 minutes or until firm enough to handle.
3 Dust the work surface with the flour, then shape the tuna and potato mixture into eight even-sized cakes. Dip into the egg white, then coat in the breadcrumbs or oats. Place on a baking sheet and cook in a preheated oven at 200°C (400°F) mark 6 for 10–15 minutes or until hot and crisp.
4 Meanwhile, mix the remaining yogurt and dill with the mayonnaise. Serve this sauce in a separate bowl with the cooked fish cakes. Garnish the fish cakes with lemon wedges and fresh dill.

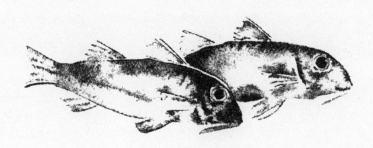

*D*EVILLED POACHED EGGS

If you own an egg poacher, use it to cook the eggs in step 4. Grease lightly with a little low-fat spread.

Serves 4

190 kcals per serving

15 ml (1 tbsp) vegetable oil
1 small onion, skinned and finely
   chopped
6 tomatoes, seeded and chopped
75 g (3 oz) button mushrooms,
   chopped
5 ml (1 tsp) whole grain mustard
15 ml (1 tbsp) tomato purée

15 ml (1 tbsp) Worcestershire sauce
200 ml (7 fl oz) chicken stock
few drops of Tabasco sauce
salt and freshly ground pepper
5 ml (1 tsp) vinegar
4 eggs
4 slices of wholemeal bread
low-fat spread, to serve

1 Heat the oil in a heavy-based saucepan. Add the onion and cook for 5 minutes or until soft. Add the tomatoes and mushrooms and simmer for a further 3 minutes.

2 Stir in the mustard, tomato purée, Worcestershire sauce, stock, Tabasco sauce and salt and pepper to taste. Simmer gently for 10–15 minutes.

3 If a smooth sauce is desired, leave to cool slightly, then purée in a blender or food processor for a few seconds. Return to the saucepan and keep hot.

4 Half-fill a large frying pan with water and bring to a rapid boil. Add the vinegar. Crack the eggs very carefully, one at a time, into a cup, then slide them into the boiling water. Poach gently until cooked to your liking.

5 Meanwhile, toast the bread and spread with a little low-fat spread. Drain the poached eggs one at a time on a perforated fish slice or slotted spoon and place an egg on each slice of toast. Spoon the hot sauce over and serve immediately.

Opposite: Chicken and Prawn Gumbo (page 25)
Overleaf: Steamed Mussels in Pepper Broth (page 30)

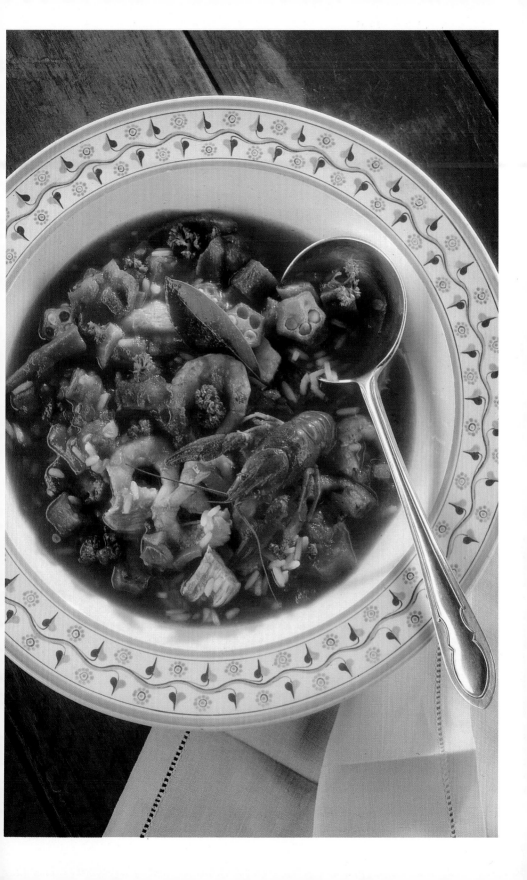

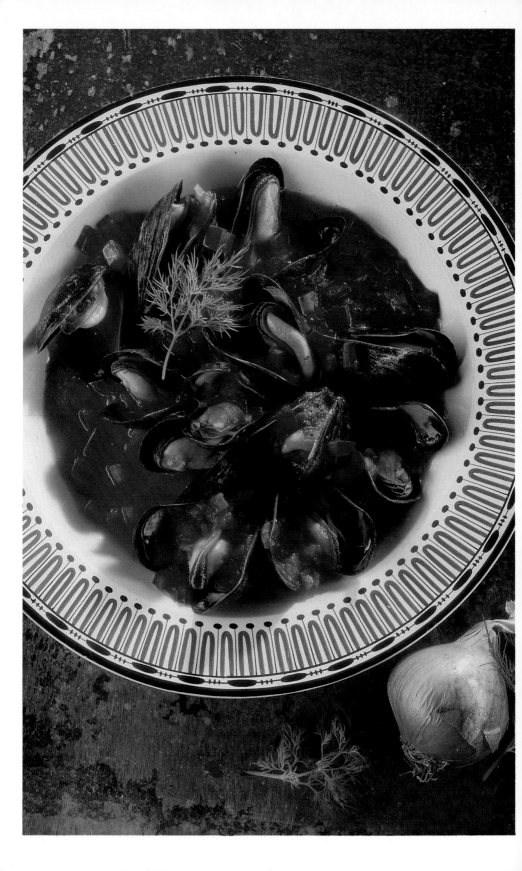

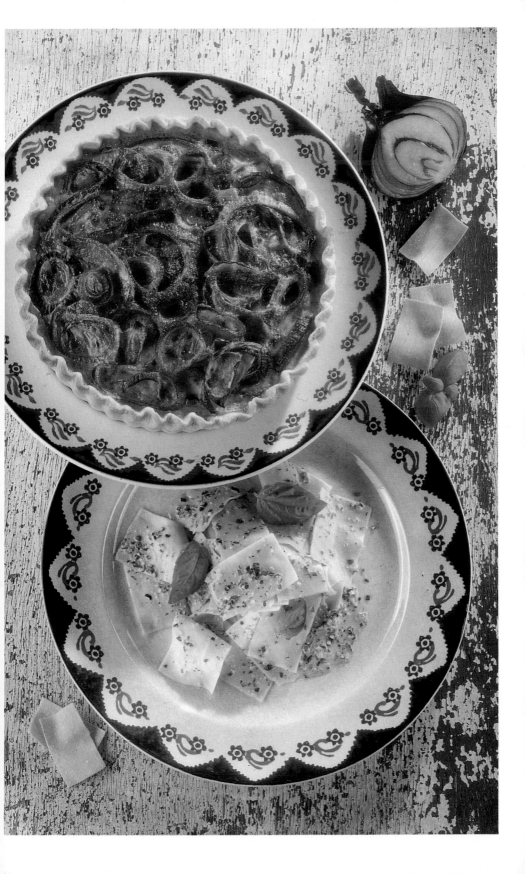

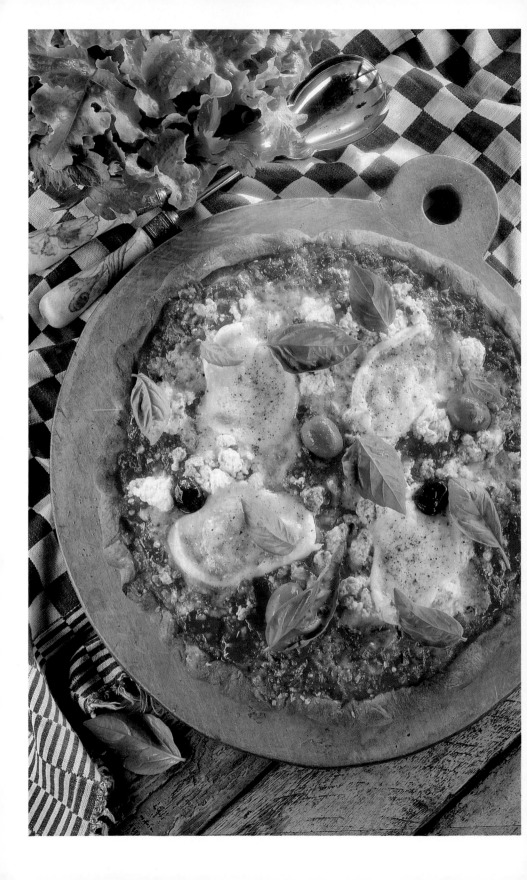

PERSIAN OMELETTE

All this substantial omelette needs as an accompaniment is crusty bread and a simple green salad tossed with a little reduced-calorie vinaigrette dressing.

Serves 4

233 kcals per serving

450 g (1 lb) fresh spinach or one
   226 g (8 oz) packet frozen
  chopped spinach
225 g (8 oz) potatoes, peeled
25 ml (1½ tbsp) vegetable oil
1 medium onion, skinned and
  chopped

4 eggs, beaten
salt and freshly ground pepper
grated rind of ½ lemon
juice of 1 lemon
15 g (½ oz) low-fat spread

1 If using fresh spinach, wash, and while still wet, place in a saucepan. Cover and cook gently for 5 minutes or until tender. Drain well and chop finely.

2 If using frozen spinach, place in a saucepan and cook for 7–10 minutes to thaw and to drive off as much liquid as possible.

3 Cut the potatoes into small dice. Heat the oil in a 20.5 cm (8 inch) non-stick frying pan, add the potato and fry gently for 5 minutes or until just turning brown. Add the onion and cook for about 10 minutes or until golden. The potato should be almost tender. Remove from the heat and set aside.

4 In a large bowl, mix the spinach with the eggs, salt and pepper to taste, lemon rind and juice. Add the potato and onion and mix well.

5 Heat the low-fat spread in the same frying pan and pour in the egg mixture, spreading it evenly over the bottom of the pan. Cover with a lid or foil and cook gently for 15 minutes or until just set.

6 Remove the lid or foil and brown the omelette under a hot grill before serving warm.

Opposite: Four-Cheese Pizza (page 40)
Previous page: Red Onion Tart (page 41); Pasta with Pesto (page 39)

CHICKEN AND PRAWN KEBABS

Serve this quick, easy supper dish with a simple pilaff made from a mixture of wild and long grain rice, green beans and lots of fresh herbs.

Serves 2

219 kcals per serving

2 chicken breast fillets, skinned
8 raw jumbo prawns
30 ml (2 tbsp) soy sauce
45 ml (3 tbsp) dry sherry
1 garlic clove, skinned and crushed
2.5 cm (1 inch) piece of fresh root
  ginger, peeled and chopped

2 spring onions, trimmed and
  chopped
1 small onion, peeled and quartered
finely shredded spring onions, to
  garnish

1 Cut the chicken into bite-sized pieces. Peel the prawns, leaving the tail shell attached. Remove the vein from down the middle of each prawn.
2 Mix the soy sauce, sherry, garlic, ginger and chopped spring onions together in a shallow dish. Add the prawns and chicken, cover and leave to marinate in a cool place overnight.
3 Thread the chicken, prawns and onion quarters on to four kebab skewers. Cook under a preheated hot grill for 10–15 minutes or until the chicken is tender, basting with the marinade and turning occasionally. Serve immediately, garnished with the spring onion shreds.

SOUFFLÉED RAREBITS

Easy to make, these are a delicious variation of the traditional Welsh rarebit, with a delightful piquant taste.

Serves 4

237 kcals per serving

4 slices of wholemeal bread
15 g (½ oz) low-fat spread, plus a little
  extra for spreading
15 ml (1 tbsp) poppy seeds
15 ml (1 tbsp) plain flour
150 ml (¼ pint) semi-skimmed milk
5 ml (1 tsp) Dijon mustard

5 ml (1 tsp) Worcestershire sauce
100 g (4 oz) Edam or Gouda cheese,
  grated
2 eggs, separated
tomato wedges and watercress
  sprigs, to garnish

1 Spread the slices of bread lightly with low-fat spread. Sprinkle each slice with poppy seeds and bake in a preheated oven at 190°C (375°F) mark 5 for 5 minutes.

2 Melt 15 g (½ oz) low-fat spread in a saucepan, stir in the flour and cook for 1 minute. Gradually stir in the milk and bring to the boil. Stir over a low heat until the sauce has thickened. Remove from the heat.

3 Beat in the mustard, Worcestershire sauce, grated cheese and egg yolks.

4 Whisk the egg whites until stiff, then fold into the cheese mixture.

5 Spoon the mixture on top of each slice of bread and return to the oven for a further 15 minutes or until puffed and golden. Serve immediately, garnished with tomato wedges and watercress sprigs.

*B*EEF KEBABS WITH HORSERADISH SAUCE

Look out for extra lean minced beef in your supermarket. It can contain as little as 10 per cent fat.

Serves 6

332 kcals per serving

700 g (1½ lb) lean minced beef
250 g (9 oz) grated onion
135 ml (9 tbsp) horseradish sauce
30 ml (2 tbsp) chopped fresh thyme
250 g (9 oz) fresh breadcrumbs
salt and freshly ground pepper

1 egg, beaten
plain flour, for coating
150 ml (5 fl oz) low-fat natural yogurt
120 ml (8 tbsp) finely chopped fresh
  parsley

1 Put the minced beef in a large bowl and mix in the onion, 90 ml (6 tbsp) of the horseradish, the thyme, breadcrumbs and salt and pepper to taste.

2 Add enough egg to bind the mixture together and, with well-floured hands, shape into 18 even-sized sausages.

3 Thread the kebabs lengthways on to six oiled kebab skewers. Place under a preheated grill and cook for about 20 minutes, turning frequently.

4 Meanwhile, mix the yogurt with the remaining horseradish and the parsley. Serve the kebabs hot, accompanied by the sauce.

CHICKEN AND WALNUT-STUFFED ONIONS WITH CHEESE SAUCE

The onion centres can be used in salads or sandwich fillings if they are chopped, wrapped tightly and stored in the refrigerator.

Serves 4

250 kcals per serving

4 large Spanish onions, each
   weighing about 275 g (10 oz),
   skinned
50 g (2 oz) long grain rice
150 g (5 oz) cooked chicken meat,
   skinned and finely chopped
50 g (2 oz) walnuts, finely chopped
15 ml (1 tbsp) lemon juice
5 ml (1 tsp) ground coriander
5 ml (1 tsp) mixed dried herbs
salt and freshly ground pepper

For the Cheese Sauce
5 ml (1 tsp) instant vegetable stock
   granules
10 ml (2 tsp) cornflour
150 ml ($\frac{1}{4}$ pint) semi-skimmed milk
30 ml (2 tbsp) low-fat soft cheese
50 g (2 oz) low-fat Cheshire cheese,
   grated
5 ml (1 tsp) ground coriander
30 ml (2 tbsp) chopped fresh parsley

1 Place the onions in a large saucepan, cover with water and bring to the boil. Lower the heat and simmer for 20 minutes. Meanwhile, cook the rice in boiling water for about 12 minutes or until tender. Drain and set aside. Drain the onions, reserving the cooking water. Set aside to cool slightly.

2 Mix together the chicken, rice, walnuts, lemon juice, coriander, herbs and salt and pepper to taste.

3 Scoop out and discard a spoonful of the centre of each onion. Stuff the centre of each onion with the chicken and walnut filling.

4 Place the onions in a casserole or ovenproof serving dish large enough to hold them upright and add 600 ml (1 pint) of the reserved cooking liquid. Cover and cook in a preheated oven at 190°C (375°F) mark 5 for $1\frac{1}{2}$ hours, basting occasionally. Drain the juices into a saucepan and keep the onions hot.

5 To make the sauce, stir the vegetable stock granules into the onion cooking juices and simmer until reduced to 150 ml ($\frac{1}{4}$ pint). Mix the cornflour with the milk and add to the pan. Bring slowly to the boil, stirring continuously, and cook for 2 minutes. Reduce the heat and stir in the cheeses, coriander and parsley. Cook very gently for 5 minutes, then pour over the onions and serve.

BUCKWHEAT NOODLES WITH CRISP VEGETABLES

Buckwheat noodles or spaghetti make a delicious alternative to whole-wheat noodles. They are available from health food shops.

Serves 4

245 kcals per serving

225 g (8 oz) buckwheat noodles or spaghetti
5 ml (1 tsp) vegetable oil
2 onions, skinned and thinly sliced
100 g (4 oz) carrots, scrubbed and thinly sliced
450 g (1 lb) mixed fresh vegetables, such as turnips, mushrooms, cabbage, fennel, peppers, swedes or broccoli florets, prepared and thinly sliced
75 g (3 oz) frozen or fresh peas or mange-tout
15 ml (1 tbsp) soy sauce
15 ml (1 tbsp) dry sherry
chilli sauce (optional)

1 Cook the noodles or spaghetti according to the instructions on the packet and drain well.
2 Heat the oil in a large frying pan or wok. Add the onions and carrots and cook over a medium heat for 5 minutes, stirring occasionally, until the onions are soft.
3 Add the remaining vegetables, soy sauce and 30 ml (2 tbsp) water. Raise the heat and cover the pan when the mixture begins to sizzle. Cook gently for 5 minutes, stirring occasionally.
4 Add the noodles, sherry and chilli sauce, if using. Stir the mixture over a medium heat for 2–3 minutes to reheat the noodles. Serve at once.

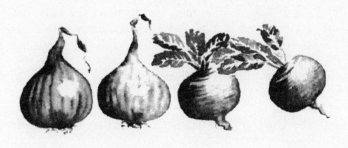

*L*EEK PANCAKES WITH WATERCRESS AND ANCHOVY SAUCE

These flavoursome pancakes need only a mixed green salad for accompaniment.

Makes 8

171 kcals per pancake

100 g (4 oz) plain flour
1 egg
300 ml (½ pint) semi-skimmed milk
salt and freshly ground pepper
15 ml (1 tbsp) snipped fresh chives
15 ml (1 tbsp) vegetable oil
25 g (1 oz) low-fat spread
3 leeks, trimmed and cut into thin
   strips
100 g (4 oz) button mushrooms,
   sliced
30 ml (2 tbsp) chopped fresh
   parsley

15 ml (1 tbsp) chopped sunflower
   seeds
50 g (2 oz) Edam cheese, grated

For the Watercress and Anchovy
   Sauce
1 bunch of watercress, chopped
4 anchovy fillets, well drained
10 ml (2 tsp) capers
30 ml (2 tbsp) olive oil
1 garlic clove, skinned and crushed
grated rind and juice of ½ lemon
about 45 ml (3 tbsp) vegetable stock

1 Put the flour into a bowl and make a well in the centre, then add the egg and half the milk and beat until smooth. Beat in the remaining milk, season with salt and pepper to taste and add the chives.

2 Lightly grease an 18 cm (7 inch) frying pan or crêpe pan with the vegetable oil, tilting the pan to coat the base and sides. Pour off any surplus oil.

3 Pour in just enough batter to coat the base of the pan. Cook for 1–2 minutes or until the underside is light brown, then turn the pancake and cook the other side. Repeat to make eight pancakes.

4 Melt the low-fat spread in a small, heavy-based saucepan and cook the leeks for about 5 minutes or until soft. Add the mushrooms and cook for a further 2 minutes, then stir in the parsley, sunflower seeds and salt and pepper to taste.

5 Lay the pancakes out flat and divide the leek filling between them, then roll up. Arrange the pancakes in a single layer in a greased shallow ovenproof dish.

6 To make the sauce, put the watercress, anchovy fillets, capers and half the olive oil in a blender or food processor and purée until smooth. Gradually blend in the remaining olive oil, the garlic, lemon rind and juice. Add enough vegetable stock to give a smooth pouring consistency. Transfer to a saucepan and heat through gently.

7   Pour the sauce over the pancakes and sprinkle with the cheese. Bake in a preheated oven at 190°C (375°F) mark 5 for 20 minutes or until heated through and golden brown.

*P*ASTA WITH PESTO

A reduced-fat version of pesto sauce is made by mixing the basic sauce with low-fat curd cheese.

Serves 4

353 kcals per serving

225 g (8 oz) pasta
30 ml (2 tbsp) olive oil
1–2 garlic cloves, skinned
about 7 g (¼ oz) fresh basil leaves
   and stems
50 g (2 oz) pine nuts

25 g (1 oz) Parmesan cheese, grated
semi-skimmed milk, to blend
100 g (4 oz) low-fat curd cheese
freshly ground pepper
fresh basil, to garnish

1   Cook the pasta in a large saucepan of boiling water for 10–12 minutes or until just tender.

2   Meanwhile, make the pesto. Put the oil, garlic, basil, pine nuts and Parmesan cheese in a blender or food processor. Add a little milk to moisten the mixture and blend to a thick purée. Transfer the purée to a bowl and stir in the curd cheese and pepper to taste.

3   Drain the pasta, return to the pan and stir in the pesto. Cook, stirring, for 1–2 minutes over a very low heat. Thin the sauce with a little more milk, if needed. Serve at once, garnished with basil.

*F*OUR-CHEESE PIZZA

Four types of Italian cheese make a pizza rich in protein, calcium and vitamins. It is quite high in calories, so serve with a large mixed salad dressed lightly with a little low-calorie dressing.

Serves 6

294 kcals per serving

5 ml (1 tsp) sugar
5 ml (1 tsp) dried yeast
100 g (4 oz) plain flour
100 g (4 oz) strong plain white flour
5 ml (1 tsp) salt
10 ml (2 tsp) vegetable oil
a few olives
fresh basil leaves, to garnish

For the Tomato Sauce
400 g (14 oz) can chopped tomatoes
5 ml (1 tsp) dried oregano

15 ml (1 tbsp) tomato purée
freshly ground pepper

For the Cheese Topping
100 g (4 oz) Mozzarella cheese, thinly
  sliced
50 g (2 oz) Docelatte cheese,
  chopped
100 g (4 oz) ricotta cheese, crumbled
30 ml (2 tbsp) grated Parmesan
  cheese

1 Lightly grease a baking sheet and set aside. To make the dough, dissolve the sugar in 150 ml (¼ pint) tepid water. Sprinkle over the yeast. Leave in a warm place for about 15 minutes or until frothy.
2 Mix the flours and salt in a bowl. Add the yeast liquid and oil. Mix to a soft dough. Turn the dough on to a floured surface and knead for 5 minutes. Return the dough to the bowl and cover with a clean cloth. Leave to rise in a warm place for 30 minutes or until doubled in size.
3 Meanwhile, place all the sauce ingredients in a saucepan, adding pepper to taste, and bring to the boil. Reduce the heat and simmer, uncovered, for 15–20 minutes or until the sauce is thick and pulpy. Remove from the heat and leave to cool.
4 Quickly knead the risen dough, then roll out to a 25 cm (10 inch) round and place on the prepared baking sheet. Fold up the edges of the dough slightly to form a rim.
5 Spread the sauce over the dough to within 1 cm (½ inch) of the edge. Arrange the Mozzarella, Dolcelatte and ricotta cheeses evenly over the sauce. Finish with a topping of Parmesan cheese. Sprinkle with the olives.
6 Bake the pizza in a preheated oven at 200°C (400°F) mark 6 for 25–30 minutes or until the cheese has melted and the dough is golden brown. Serve the pizza piping hot, garnished with basil leaves.

*R*ED ONION TART

Red onions are slightly oval shaped and smaller than globe onions. They have a mild, somewhat sweet flavour.

Serves 8

207 kcals per serving

175 g (6 oz) plain flour
75 g (3 oz) margarine or butter
15 ml (1 tbsp) vegetable oil
4 red onions, skinned and thinly sliced

75 ml (5 tbsp) semi-skimmed milk
3 eggs
2.5 ml (½ tsp) cayenne

1 Put the flour into a mixing bowl and rub in the margarine or butter until the mixture resembles fine breadcrumbs. Mix to a firm but pliable dough with about 30 ml (2 tbsp) cold water. Knead on a lightly floured surface.
2 Roll out the dough and use to line a 20.5 cm (8 inch) loose-based flan tin. Chill for 30 minutes.
3 Place a sheet of greaseproof paper in the base of the flan case, cover with baking beans and bake blind in a preheated oven at 200°C (400°F) mark 6 for 15 minutes. Remove the beans and paper, then bake for a further 5 minutes.
4 Meanwhile, heat the oil in a heavy-based saucepan, add the onions, cover and cook for 6–8 minutes or until transparent. Drain off the oil, then place the onions in the partially baked flan case.
5 Beat the milk with the eggs and cayenne. Pour into the partially baked flan case and bake for 25–30 minutes or until the filling is set and golden. Serve immediately.

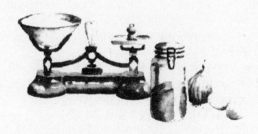

SPINACH AND CHEESE PIE WITH POTATO CRUST

The potato crust can be prepared in advance and stored, covered, in the refrigerator.

Makes 6 slices

120 kcals per slice

275 g (10 oz) trimmed spinach
leaves, finely shredded
3 eggs
225 g (8 oz) ricotta cheese
100 g (4 oz) low-fat soft cheese
30 ml (2 tbsp) grated Parmesan
cheese
5 ml (1 tsp) grated nutmeg
finely grated rind of 1 lemon
juice of ½ lemon
freshly ground pepper

50 ml (2 fl oz) semi-skimmed milk
paprika, for sprinkling

For the Crisp Potato Crust
100 g (4 oz) plain flour
50 g (2 oz) margarine or butter
100 g (4 oz) potatoes, scrubbed and
finely grated
½ small onion, skinned and grated
salt and freshly ground pepper
5 ml (1 tsp) vegetable oil

1   To make the crust, put the flour in a bowl and rub in the margarine or butter until the mixture resembles fine breadcrumbs. Squeeze the grated potatoes well, to remove as much excess moisture as possible, then add to the flour mixture with the onion and salt and pepper to taste. Mix to a firm dough.
2   With lightly floured fingers, thinly press the dough over the base and sides of a 20.5 cm (8 inch) flan tin or dish. Bake in a preheated oven at 200°C (400°F) mark 6 for 20 minutes. Brush with the oil and bake for a further 10 minutes or until the crust is crisp.
3   Meanwhile, place the spinach in a steamer or colander over boiling water. Cover tightly and steam for 1 minute or until just tender. Set aside.
4   Beat together the eggs, ricotta cheese, low-fat soft cheese, half the Parmesan cheese, the nutmeg, lemon rind and juice, pepper to taste and milk until smooth. Add the spinach and mix gently.
5   Reduce the oven temperature to 180°C (350°F) mark 4. Spoon the spinach and cheese mixture into the cooked crust and level the surface. Sprinkle over the remaining Parmesan cheese and the paprika. Bake for 30–35 minutes or until lightly coloured and set. Serve warm or cold.

*C*HILLI, AUBERGINE AND RED PEPPER SALAD

Serve this unusual smoky flavoured salad with hot pitta bread to make a complete lunch or supper.

Serves 4

131 kcals per serving

2 red peppers
3 medium aubergines, about 700 g (1½ lb) total weight
salt and freshly ground pepper
30 ml (2 tbsp) olive or vegetable oil
2 medium onions, skinned and roughly chopped
15 ml (1 tbsp) chilli seasoning

1.25 ml (¼ tsp) chilli powder
150 ml (¼ pint) dry white wine
30 ml (2 tbsp) tomato purée
15 ml (1 tbsp) lemon juice
15 ml (1 tbsp) wine vinegar
2.5 ml (½ tsp) granulated sugar
chopped fresh parsley, to garnish

1 Put the whole red peppers under a preheated moderate grill and turn them constantly until their skins are charred all over. Put the peppers in a bowl.
2 Trim the aubergines and cut into 2.5 cm (1 inch) cubes. Place in a colander, sprinkling each layer with salt. Cover with a plate, put heavy weights on top and leave to dégorge for about 30 minutes.
3 Meanwhile, hold the peppers under cold running water and rub the skins off with your fingers. Discard the skins, stems, cores and seeds. Cut the pepper flesh into long, thin shreds and place in a serving bowl.
4 Rinse the aubergines under cold running water, then pat dry with absorbent kitchen paper. Heat the oil in a heavy-based saucepan. Add the aubergines and onions and fry over moderate heat for 3–4 minutes. Stir in the chilli seasoning and powder. Fry for 1–2 minutes, then add the wine, tomato purée, lemon juice, vinegar, sugar and salt and pepper to taste.
5 Bring to the boil, cover and simmer for 10–12 minutes or until the aubergine is cooked. Leave to cool for 30 minutes, then add to the pepper strips in the serving bowl.
6 Cover the salad and chill in the refrigerator for 1 hour. Sprinkle with plenty of chopped parsley before serving.

*H*OT SPICED CHICK-PEA SALAD

A very quick supper dish to make from storecupboard ingredients. Serve with crusty wholemeal bread.

Serves 4

345 kcals per serving

15 ml (1 tbsp) vegetable oil
1 medium onion, skinned and roughly chopped
10 ml (2 tsp) ground turmeric
15 ml (1 tbsp) cumin seeds
450 g (1 lb) tomatoes, roughly chopped

two 400 g (14 oz) cans cooked chick-peas, drained
15 ml (1 tbsp) lemon juice
60 ml (4 tbsp) chopped fresh coriander
salt and freshly ground pepper
coriander leaves, to garnish

1 Heat the oil in a medium saucepan and sauté the onion for about 10 minutes or until golden brown.
2 Add the turmeric and cumin seeds and cook, stirring, for 1–2 minutes before adding the remaining ingredients, except the coriander leaves.
3 Continue cooking for 1–2 minutes, stirring frequently. Adjust the seasoning and serve garnished with fresh coriander leaves.

*F*RESH FISH AND SHELLFISH

*F*ISH has both a low saturated fat content and a low calorie content. It's a good source of protein and can be cooked quickly, in an endless number of ways. For some reason, however, many people have an aversion to fresh fish, thinking it difficult and time-consuming to prepare. It is frequently shunned in favour of frozen and pre-cooked fish products which are often unnecessarily loaded with fat, preservatives and colourings that successfully mask the true taste of fish. Get your fishmonger to clean, fillet and skin fish, or look for it ready-prepared in larger supermarkets – you won't be disappointed by the taste of the real thing.

When buying fish and shellfish, look for clear, bright eyes, bright red or pink gills, shiny, firm bodies and firmly attached scales. Fillets, steaks and cutlets should be firm and moist and not show any sign of dryness or discoloration. They should not be wet and slimy. Shellfish should have tightly closed and undamaged shells. All fish and shellfish should smell of the sea – not fishy!

The healthiest, lowest-calorie methods of cooking fish are poaching, grilling, steaming, baking or microwaving. Fish products that are coated in batter, then deep-fried, soak up lots of fat. Coat in egg and breadcrumbs instead and bake in the oven. If buying commercially-prepared fish products, check packets for brands suitable for oven-baking. For some more interesting ways to enhance the naturally delicious flavour of fresh fish and shellfish, simply read through the recipes in this chapter.

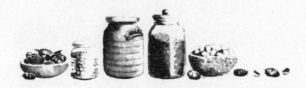

*L*EMON SOLE IN LETTUCE

Don't overcook the lettuce in step 1, or the dish will be ruined. The leaves should be dropped into the water and then removed almost immediately.

Serves 4

220 kcals per serving

16 large lettuce leaves, thick stalks removed
8 fillets of lemon sole, each weighing about 100 g (4 oz), skinned
15 ml (1 tbsp) lemon juice
salt and freshly ground pepper

100 g (4 oz) peeled cooked prawns, thawed if frozen
15 ml (1 tbsp) chopped fresh dill
150 ml (¼ pint) fish stock or dry white wine
lemon slices, to garnish

1   Drop the lettuce leaves into a large saucepan of boiling water and simmer for 1 minute. Drain and rinse in cold water until the leaves are chilled. Dry on absorbent kitchen paper, then spread out on a flat surface.

2   Sprinkle the fillets with a little of the lemon juice and season with salt and pepper to taste. Arrange a few prawns in the centre of each fillet and sprinkle over half the dill. Fold the fish into thirds to enclose the prawns.

3   Place each folded fillet on a lettuce leaf and roll up again, folding the edges to form a neat parcel.

4   Place the fish parcels in a non-stick frying pan and sprinkle over the remaining lemon juice, stock or wine and pepper to taste. Cover and cook gently for 15 minutes or until tender.

5   Remove the fish to a warmed serving dish. Boil the cooking juices until reduced to about 90 ml (6 tbsp). Stir in the remaining dill and pour over the fish. Serve garnished with lemon slices.

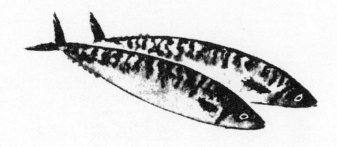

MINT AND MACKEREL PARCELS

Fillet the mackerel yourself, as instructed here, or get your fishmonger to do it for you.

Serves 4

232 kcals per serving

4 fresh mackerel, each weighing about 175 g (6 oz)
about 25 g (1 oz) low-fat spread
½ large cucumber, thinly sliced
60 ml (4 tbsp) white wine vinegar

30 ml (2 tbsp) chopped fresh mint
5 ml (1 tsp) sugar
salt and freshly ground pepper
low-fat natural yogurt and chopped fresh mint, to serve

1 With the back of a knife and working from the tail towards the head, scrape off the scales from the skin of the mackerel.
2 Cut off the heads just below the gills with a sharp knife. Cut off the fins and tails with kitchen scissors.
3 Slit open the underside of each fish, from head to tail end, with a sharp knife or scissors. With the flat of the knife blade, scrape out the entrails of the fish, together with any membranes and blood. Wash the fish thoroughly inside and out under cold running water.
4 Open out each fish and lay it flat on a board or work surface with the skin uppermost. Press firmly along the backbone with your knuckles (this flattens the fish and loosens the backbone).
5 Turn the fish over and lift out the backbone with the help of a knife. Cut each fish lengthways into two fillets. Dry thoroughly with absorbent kitchen paper.
6 Spread eight squares of kitchen foil with a little low-fat spread. Put a mackerel fillet in the centre of each square, skin-side down.
7 Arrange cucumber slices down one half of the length of each mackerel fillet, then sprinkle with the vinegar, mint, sugar and salt and pepper to taste. Dot with tiny pieces of the remaining low-fat spread.
8 Fold the mackerel fillets over lengthways to enclose the cucumber filling, then wrap in the foil. Place the foil parcels in a single layer in an ovenproof dish. Cook in a preheated oven at 200°C (400°F) mark 6 for 30 minutes or until the fish is tender.
9 To serve, unwrap the foil parcels and carefully place the mackerel fillets on a warmed platter. Spoon over the yogurt and sprinkle with the chopped mint.

*M*ARINATED TROUT WITH FENNEL

The bulb vegetable Florence fennel looks rather like a squat version of celery with feathery leaves. The flavour of fennel is like aniseed. For the most subtle taste of aniseed, buy white or pale green fennel; for a stronger flavour, choose vegetables which are dark green in colour.

Serves 4

221 kcals per serving

30 ml (2 tbsp) olive oil
4 whole trout, each weighing about
   225 g (8 oz), cleaned
30 ml (2 tbsp) plain flour
1 small bulb Florence fennel, trimmed
   and finely sliced

1 onion, skinned and finely sliced
300 ml (½ pint) dry white wine
finely grated rind and juice of
   1 orange
salt and freshly ground pepper
orange slices, to garnish

1   Heat the olive oil in a frying pan. Dip the trout in the flour and fry gently for 4 minutes on each side. With a fish slice, transfer the fish to a shallow dish.

2   With a sharp knife, score the skin of the trout diagonally, being careful not to cut too deeply into the flesh. Set aside.

3   Add the fennel and onion to the frying pan and fry for 5 minutes. Add the wine, orange rind and juice, and salt and pepper to taste. Bring to the boil and boil rapidly for 1 minute. Pour immediately over the fish. Leave to cool.

4   Place the trout in the refrigerator and leave to marinate for at least 8 hours, but no more than 3 days.

5   Serve at room temperature, garnished with orange slices.

SPANISH COD WITH PEPPERS, TOMATOES AND GARLIC

This substantial meal-in-one fish dish is ideal for a family supper. Serve with hot French bread.

Serves 4

293 kcals per serving

1.1 litres (1¾ pints) fresh mussels, or about 450 g (1 lb) in weight
salt and freshly ground pepper
a little oatmeal
700 g (1½ lb) cod fillets, skinned
15 ml (1 tbsp) vegetable oil
2 onions, skinned and sliced
1 red pepper, cored, seeded and sliced

1 green pepper, cored, seeded and sliced
1–2 garlic cloves, skinned and crushed
450 g (1 lb) tomatoes, skinned and chopped
300 ml (½ pint) white wine
2.5 ml (½ tsp) Tabasco sauce
1 bay leaf

1 Discard any cracked mussels and any that remain open when tapped sharply on the shell. Scrub the mussels, pull off the coarse threads (beards) from the sides of the shells and soak in cold water, with a little salt and oatmeal added, for at least 30 minutes or overnight.
2 Using a sharp knife, cut the cod into chunks.
3 Drain and rinse the mussels and place in a large saucepan. Cover and cook over a high heat for about 8 minutes or until all the mussels have opened. Discard any that do not open.
4 Shell all but a handful of the mussels. Heat the oil in a heavy-based frying pan and cook the onions, peppers and garlic for about 5 minutes or until starting to soften. Add the tomatoes and wine, bring to the boil and simmer for 5 minutes, then add the Tabasco.
5 Layer the fish and vegetables in a casserole and add the bay leaf and salt and pepper to taste. Pour over the wine. Push the reserved mussels in their shells into the top layer. Cover and cook in a preheated oven at 180°C (350°F) mark 4 for 1 hour. Serve hot.

RED MULLET BAKED IN PAPER

Red mullet is known as the woodcock of the sea because you can eat it all – there's no need to remove the insides. Cooking in paper conserves all the juices, and the parcels, when opened at the table, show the attractive red colour to advantage as well as allowing diners to enjoy the delicious smell as the paper is opened.

Serves 2

350 kcals per serving

2 red mullet, each weighing about 225 g (8 oz)
15 ml (1 tbsp) chopped fresh parsley
1 small onion, skinned and sliced
50 g (2 oz) mushrooms, chopped
finely grated rind and juice of 1 lemon
salt and freshly ground pepper

1 Cut two squares of greaseproof paper, each large enough to wrap one fish. Place the fish on top, then add half the remaining ingredients to each fish. Fold the paper to make secure parcels.
2 Place the parcels on a baking sheet and bake in a preheated oven at 180°C (350°F) mark 4 for 30 minutes or until the fish is tender. Serve the fish in their parcels.

WATERCRESS-STUFFED PLAICE

Serve with lightly steamed mange-tout or green beans and new potatoes.

Serves 4

315 kcals per serving

15 g (½ oz) low-fat spread
1 small onion, skinned and finely chopped
1 bunch of watercress, trimmed and finely chopped
75 g (3 oz) fresh breadcrumbs
finely grated rind of 1 small lemon
50 g (2 oz) Mozzarella cheese, grated
salt and freshly ground pepper
30 ml (2 tbsp) beaten egg
8 plaice fillets, each weighing about 100 g (4 oz), skinned
30 ml (2 tbsp) lemon juice
75 ml (3 fl oz) vegetable stock, dry white wine or water
watercress, to garnish

1 Lightly grease a shallow ovenproof dish and set aside. Melt the low-fat spread in a small saucepan, add the onion and watercress and cook gently for 5 minutes, stirring occasionally. Stir in the breadcrumbs, lemon rind and cheese. Season with salt and pepper to taste and bind the mixture with the egg.

2 Put the plaice fillets, skinned sides upwards, on a board. Sprinkle with salt and pepper to taste and cover the tail end half of each fillet with stuffing. Fold over the remaining half fillet to form a neat parcel.

3 Arrange the stuffed fillets in the prepared dish. Sprinkle with the lemon juice and stock, wine or water. Cover with foil and cook in a pre-heated oven at 190°C (375°F) mark 5 for 25 minutes or until tender.

*C*EVICHE

Ceviche is a Mexican dish of raw fish marinated in lime juice. The acid 'cooks' the fish. Don't be put off by the idea of raw fish – it is delicious.

Serves 4

148 kcals per serving

700 g (1½ lb) haddock fillets, skinned
15 ml (1 tbsp) coriander seeds
5 ml (1 tsp) black peppercorns
juice of 6 limes
5 ml (1 tsp) salt
1 hot chilli, seeded and chopped
1 bunch of spring onions, trimmed
   and sliced
4 tomatoes, skinned and chopped

1 small red pepper, cored, seeded
   and thinly sliced
few drops of Tabasco sauce, or to
   taste
45 ml (3 tbsp) chopped fresh
   coriander
salt and freshly ground pepper
lime slices and fresh coriander, to
   garnish

1 Cut the fish fillets diagonally into thin, even strips and place in a bowl.

2 Crush the coriander seeds and peppercorns to a fine powder in a pestle and mortar. Mix with the lime juice, 5 ml (1 tsp) salt and the chilli, then pour over the fish. Cover and chill in the refrigerator for 24 hours, turning the fish occasionally.

3 To serve, drain the fish from the marinade, discarding the marinade. Mix the fish with the remaining ingredients, seasoning with salt and pepper to taste, if necessary. Serve chilled, garnished with lime slices and coriander leaves.

SPICED GRILLED HALIBUT

The flavours of India transform everyday halibut in this spicy grilled fish dish. Cod or haddock could also be treated in this way.

Serves 4

190 kcals per serving

4 halibut steaks, each weighing about 175 g (6 oz)
75 ml (5 tbsp) low-fat natural yogurt
2 garlic cloves, skinned and crushed
1 onion, skinned and finely chopped
15 ml (1 tbsp) paprika
5 ml (1 tsp) garam masala
5 ml (1 tsp) ground coriander
5 ml (1 tsp) ground cumin

salt and freshly ground pepper
2.5 ml (½ tsp) ground turmeric
1 red chilli, seeded and finely chopped
5 ml (1 tsp) grated fresh root ginger
juice of 1 lemon
lemon wedges and chopped fresh coriander, to garnish

1 Wash the halibut steaks under cold running water, drain and then place in a large, shallow, heatproof dish.
2 Put all the remaining ingredients, except those for the garnish, into a blender or food processor and purée until smooth. Pour over the fish. Cover and leave to marinate in a cool place for 24 hours, turning occasionally.
3 Cook the fish under a preheated hot grill, basting occasionally with the marinade, until the fish flakes easily when tested with a fork.
4 Serve the fish hot, garnished with lemon wedges and coriander.

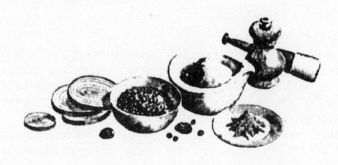

*F*ISHERMAN'S PIE

Try serving Fisherman's Pie with fresh spinach. Wash the spinach and cook for a few minutes in the water clinging to the leaves, then drain, roughly chop and lightly season with salt, pepper and grated nutmeg.

Serves 4

335 kcals per serving

50 g (2 oz) low-fat spread
100 g (4 oz) red pepper, cored, seeded and thinly sliced
100 g (4 oz) green pepper, cored, seeded and thinly sliced
50 g (2 oz) onion, skinned and sliced
salt and freshly ground pepper

100 g (4 oz) button mushrooms, halved
450 ml (¾ pint) tomato juice
550 g (1¼ lb) cod fillet, skinned
450 g (1 lb) potatoes, peeled and very thinly sliced
50 g (2 oz) Edam cheese, grated

1 Melt 25 g (1 oz) of the low-fat spread in a frying pan, add the peppers and onion and fry gently for 10 minutes or until soft but not coloured. Transfer to a 2.3 litre (4 pint) ovenproof dish. Season well with salt and pepper to taste.

2 Add the mushrooms to the frying pan and cook in the remaining fat for 3–4 minutes, stirring frequently, until evenly coloured.

3 Pour the tomato juice evenly over the pepper and onion mixture in the dish.

4 Cut the fish into large cubes. Arrange the cubes on top of the tomato juice, pressing them down gently into the juice. Top with the mushrooms. Season again with salt and pepper to taste.

5 Arrange the potato slices on top of the mushrooms. Melt the remaining low-fat spread and brush over the potatoes. Bake in a preheated oven at 190°C (375°F) mark 5 for 25 minutes.

6 Sprinkle the grated cheese over the pie, return to the oven and bake for a further 15 minutes or until melted and bubbling. Serve hot, straight from the dish.

SWEET AND SOUR FISH

This oriental dish is delicious accompanied simply by boiled rice. A 50 g (2 oz) serving of boiled rice would add an extra 70 kcals to the meal.

Serves 4

203 kcals per serving

225 g (8 oz) can pineapple slices in natural juice, drained, with juice reserved

15 ml (1 tbsp) soy sauce

60 ml (4 tbsp) red wine vinegar

30 ml (2 tbsp) sugar

15 ml (1 tbsp) tomato purée

30 ml (2 tbsp) dry sherry

30 ml (2 tbsp) cornflour

30 ml (2 tbsp) vegetable oil

1 small onion, skinned and sliced

1 red pepper, cored, seeded and thinly sliced

2 carrots, scrubbed and sliced

2.5 cm (1 inch) piece of fresh root ginger, peeled and chopped

225 g (8 oz) can water chestnuts, drained and sliced

100 g (4 oz) button mushrooms, sliced

450 g (1 lb) haddock fillet, skinned and cut into bite-sized pieces

175 g (6 oz) peeled cooked prawns, thawed if frozen

225 g (8 oz) fresh beansprouts

1 Cut each pineapple slice into chunks. Make up the reserved juice to 300 ml ($\frac{1}{2}$ pint) with water. Add the soy sauce, vinegar, sugar, tomato purée, sherry and cornflour. Mix until smooth.

2 Heat the oil in a large non-stick frying pan or wok. Add the onion, pepper, carrots and ginger and cook over a high heat for 3 minutes, stirring constantly. Add the pineapple, water chestnuts and mushrooms and stir-fry for a further 2 minutes.

3 Stir the pineapple juice mixture and add to the pan. Bring to the boil, stirring. Add the haddock and prawns and simmer for 2–3 minutes or until cooked. Stir in the beansprouts and heat through. Serve at once.

MONKFISH AND PRAWN TERRINE

This can be made in advance and stored, covered, in the refrigerator. Serve with a colourful mixed salad.

Serves 4

195 kcals per serving

450 g (1 lb) monkfish fillet, skinned
60 ml (4 tbsp) chopped fresh dill or
    30 ml (2 tbsp) dried
50 ml (2 fl oz) dry white wine
1 egg white, size 2
salt and freshly ground pepper
100 g (4 oz) peeled cooked prawns,
    thawed if frozen, chopped

1 small bunch of watercress, finely
    chopped
4 tomatoes, skinned, seeded and
    finely chopped
1 garlic clove, skinned and crushed
150 ml (5 fl oz) low-fat natural yogurt
unpeeled cooked prawns, to garnish

1 Lightly oil a 450 g (1 lb) loaf tin and set aside. Place the monkfish, chopped dill, wine, egg white and salt and pepper to taste in a blender or food processor and purée until smooth. In another bowl, mix the prawns and watercress together.

2 Spread half the monkfish purée in the base of the prepared loaf tin. Sprinkle over the prawns and watercress, then spread the remaining purée over the top. Smooth with a knife, then cover with aluminium foil.

3 Put the dish in a roasting pan with enough boiling water to come half-way up the sides. Cook in a preheated oven at 200°C (400°F) mark 6 for 45 minutes or until firm. Drain off any liquid, then leave to cool for 1 hour.

4 Meanwhile, make the tomato sauce. Put the tomatoes and garlic in a small saucepan and simmer for 10 minutes, stirring occasionally. Mix in the yogurt and season with salt and pepper to taste, then leave the mixture to cool.

5 Turn out the terrine on to a serving dish and garnish with the unpeeled cooked prawns. Cut the terrine into slices and serve with the tomato sauce.

SEAFOOD KEBABS

Monkfish is a good choice for kebabs because it retains its shape when cooked.

Serves 4

225 kcals per serving

700 g (1½ lb) monkfish or cod fillet, skinned
half a cucumber
1 lemon or lime
50 g (2 oz) large peeled cooked prawns, thawed if frozen
75 ml (3 fl oz) low-calorie vinaigrette

1 garlic clove, skinned and crushed
15 ml (1 tbsp) chopped fresh dill or 2.5 ml (½ tsp) dried
salt and freshly ground pepper
green salad and dill sprigs, to serve

1 Cut the fish into 2.5 cm (1 inch) cubes. Halve the cucumber lengthways and cut into thick slices. Thinly slice the lemon or lime.
2 Wrap a lemon or lime slice round each prawn. Thread on to eight wooden skewers, alternating with the cubes of fish and cucumber. Place the kebabs in a heatproof dish.
3 Mix the vinaigrette with the garlic and dill, then spoon over the kebabs. Cook under a preheated hot grill for 4–5 minutes on each side, basting occasionally. Season with salt and pepper to taste and serve immediately on a bed of green salad, garnished with dill sprigs.

SPICY SCALLOPS

Serve these delicious scallops on a bed of steamed, shredded Chinese leaves.

Serves 4

160 kcals per serving

350 g (12 oz) queen scallops, thawed if frozen
10 ml (2 tsp) Chinese sweet chilli sauce
100 g (4 oz) carrots, scrubbed
3 celery sticks, trimmed

15 ml (1 tbsp) dry sherry
15 ml (1 tbsp) soy sauce
5 ml (1 tsp) tomato purée
30 ml (2 tbsp) vegetable oil
5 ml (1 tsp) grated fresh root ginger
15 ml (1 tbsp) chopped spring onion

1 Mix the scallops with the chilli sauce and set aside. Cut the carrots and celery into thin matchsticks. Mix together the sherry, soy sauce and tomato purée with 30 ml (2 tbsp) water.

2 Heat half the oil in a large frying pan or wok. Add the carrot and celery and stir-fry over a high heat for 1 minute. Remove the vegetables from the pan with a slotted spoon and set aside.

3 Heat the remaining oil in the pan, then add the ginger and spring onion and stir-fry briefly over a high heat. Add the scallops and turn them in the oil to seal them on all sides.

4 Lower the heat to medium, add the soy sauce mixture to the pan and stir well. Return the vegetables to the pan and stir well. Stir-fry for 2–3 minutes or until the scallops feel firm. Serve immediately.

*I*NDONESIAN FISH STEW

This hearty, spicy stew needs no accompaniment other than chunks of crusty wholemeal bread.

Serves 4

220 kcals per serving

100 g (4 oz) desiccated coconut
2 large potatoes, scrubbed and cubed
4 spring onions, trimmed, with green and white parts chopped separately
finely grated rind of ½ lemon or 1 lime
salt and freshly ground pepper

1.25 ml (¼ tsp) chilli powder, or to taste (optional)
550 g (1¼ lb) white fish fillets (such as cod or haddock), skinned and cubed
2 tomatoes, cut into wedges
lemon or lime slices and coriander sprigs, to garnish

1 Put the coconut in a saucepan and add 600 ml (1 pint) water. Bring to the boil, stirring. Remove from the heat, cover and leave to cool for 20 minutes. Strain through a fine sieve into a saucepan and discard the coconut in the sieve.

2 Add the potatoes, the white parts of the spring onions, the lemon or lime rind, salt and pepper to taste and chilli powder (if using) to the coconut milk. Bring to the boil, lower the heat and simmer until the potatoes are tender but not soft.

3 Add the fish and tomatoes. Sprinkle the green spring onion parts over the top. Cover and simmer for 10 minutes or until the fish is tender. Garnish with lemon or lime slices and sprigs of coriander and serve.

*I*TALIAN SQUID STEW

Serve this rich stew with slices of French bread that have been rubbed with garlic and baked in the oven until crisp. End the meal with a refreshing sorbet or granita and fresh fruit.

Serves 4

240 kcals per serving

1 kg (2¼ lb) small squid
30 ml (2 tbsp) olive oil
salt and freshly ground pepper
150 ml (¼ pint) dry white wine

2 garlic cloves, skinned and crushed
juice of ½ lemon
45 ml (3 tbsp) chopped fresh parsley

1   Wash the squid in plenty of cold water. Grip the head and tentacles firmly and pull them away from the body. The entrails will follow. Discard these and pull out the transparent quill.

2   With your hands, carefully peel the skin from the body and the fins of the squid.

3   Cut the tentacles from the head and remove the skin. Reserve the two ink sacs, being careful not to pierce them. Discard the rest of the head.

4   Cut the squid bodies into 0.5 cm (¼ inch) rings. Place in a bowl with the tentacles, spoon over the oil and season well with salt and pepper. Leave to marinate for 3 hours.

5   Pour the squid and marinade into a large frying pan and cook for 5 minutes, turning frequently. Add the wine and garlic and cook for a further 5 minutes. Add the ink sacs, breaking them up with a spoon.

6   Cover and cook over a low heat for about 40 minutes or until the squid is tender.

7   Add the lemon juice and parsley. Stir for 3 minutes over a high heat, then adjust the seasoning and serve.

*P*ERFECT POULTRY AND GAME

*P*OULTRY is a favourite for every occasion. Available in a variety of forms, it can be cooked in many ways. Most poultry and game is healthier than red meat as it is lower in saturated fat. When buying poultry, look for a plump breast, smooth unbroken skin and a pliable breastbone tip. If it is wrapped, check that the plastic covering is unbroken. If you are buying a frozen bird, check that the bag is not damaged and that there is not an excessive amount of frozen liquid inside the bag. Game birds are best eaten young. Smooth pliable legs, short spurs and a firm, plump breast are the things to look for.

Poultry is so lean it benefits from moist forms of cooking. Poaching is ideal; it produces tender meat, without requiring the addition of any fat. Simply place the bird in a pan with enough water to cover and plenty of vegetables and a bouquet garni for flavour. For the most succulent meat, bring the water just to the boil, then reduce the heat and cook at a gentle simmer. Use the cooking liquid for sauces and soups.

Game is usually roasted covered with fatty bacon. While on a diet, it's better to casserole or braise instead. Alternatively, marinate in a strongly flavoured wine-based marinade and barbecue or grill, basting with the marinade to keep the meat moist. This chapter demonstrates the versatility of poultry and game, even within the confines of a low-calorie regime.

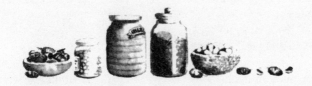

*B*AKED CHICKEN FILLETS WITH PESTO

A small baked potato served with the chicken adds 85 kcals. There's no need to put butter in the potato; the juices from the chicken add sufficient moisture. For a complete main course, serve with a mixed green salad.

Serves 4

255 kcals per serving

4 skinned chicken breast fillets, about
   450 g (1 lb) total weight
100 g (4 oz) low-fat soft cheese
30 ml (2 tbsp) bottled pesto sauce

salt and freshly ground pepper
4 thin slices of lean ham
shredded basil, to garnish

1 Make a deep horizontal cut in each chicken fillet to form a pocket.
2 Mix together the cheese and pesto and season with salt and pepper to taste. Spoon most of the mixture into the 'pockets'. Wrap each fillet with a slice of ham.
3 Place the chicken fillets on individual pieces of foil, spoon over the remaining cheese mixture and wrap in the foil.
4 Place on a baking sheet and cook in a preheated oven at 200°C (400°F) mark 6 for 25–30 minutes or until the chicken is tender.
5 Serve the chicken and juices, garnished with shredded basil.

*M*ANGO AND CHICKEN PARCELS

Use ripe mangoes, which 'give' if gently squeezed and have a sweet aroma.

Serves 4

205 kcals per serving

4 skinned chicken breast fillets, each
   weighing about 100–175 g (4–6 oz)
2 fresh mangoes
2.5 cm (1 inch) piece of fresh root
   ginger, peeled and finely chopped

freshly ground pepper
lime slices and wedges and fresh
   coriander sprigs, to garnish

1 Slash the chicken breasts vertically, but do not cut all the way through. Place on individual pieces of foil large enough to make secure parcels around the chicken.

2   Peel and remove all the flesh from the mangoes and discard the stones. Place the flesh in a bowl with the ginger and mash with a fork.

3   Spread the mango mixture evenly over the chicken and season with pepper to taste. Seal the foil around the chicken and place on a baking sheet. Cook in a preheated oven at 190°C (375°F) mark 5 for 25–30 minutes or until the chicken is cooked through. Open the parcels and garnish with the lime and coriander sprigs. Serve immediately, leaving the chicken in the foil.

STIR-FRIED CHICKEN WITH VEGETABLES AND CASHEW NUTS

With meat and vegetables cooked together, this Chinese-style dish is quite substantial. Provide extra soy sauce for those who like it.

Serves 4

195 kcals per serving

4 skinned chicken breast fillets
30 ml (2 tbsp) sesame or vegetable oil
1 bunch of spring onions, trimmed and finely sliced
3 celery sticks, trimmed and finely sliced
1 green pepper, cored, seeded and cut into thin strips
100 g (4 oz) cauliflower florets, divided into tiny sprigs

2 carrots, scrubbed and grated
175 g (6 oz) button mushrooms, finely sliced
10 ml (2 tsp) cornflour
30 ml (2 tbsp) dry sherry
15 ml (1 tbsp) soy sauce
15 ml (1 tbsp) hoisin sauce
5 ml (1 tsp) soft brown sugar
50 g (2 oz) cashew nuts
salt and freshly ground pepper

1   With a sharp knife, cut the chicken into bite-sized strips about 4 cm (1½ inches) long.

2   Heat the oil in a wok or deep frying pan, add all the prepared vegetables and stir-fry over a brisk heat for 3 minutes. Remove the vegetables with a slotted spoon and set aside.

3   In a jug, mix the cornflour to a paste with the sherry, soy sauce and hoisin sauce, then add the sugar and 150 ml (¼ pint) water.

4   Add the chicken strips to the pan and stir-fry over a moderate heat until lightly coloured on all sides. Pour the cornflour mixture into the pan and bring to the boil, stirring constantly, until thickened.

5   Return the vegetables to the pan. Add the cashew nuts and salt and pepper to taste, and stir-fry for a few minutes more. Serve immediately.

CHICKEN BAKED WITH YOGURT AND SPICES

Serve this chicken dish as an unusual alternative to the Sunday roast, accompanied by plain boiled rice.

Serves 4 or 6

359 or 239 kcals per serving

1.4 kg (3 lb) chicken
60 ml (4 tbsp) lemon or lime juice
2 garlic cloves, skinned and finely chopped
2.5 cm (1 inch) piece of fresh root ginger, peeled and finely chopped
10 ml (2 tsp) ground cumin
10 ml (2 tsp) ground coriander
5 ml (1 tsp) garam masala
10 ml (2 tsp) salt

2.5 ml (½ tsp) freshly ground pepper
30 ml (2 tbsp) vegetable oil
2 medium onions, skinned and finely sliced
5 ml (1 tsp) ground turmeric
2.5 ml (½ tsp) cayenne
300 ml (½ pint) low-fat natural yogurt
50 g (2 oz) unsalted cashew nuts or blanched almonds
chopped fresh coriander, to garnish

1 Skin the chicken completely, leaving it whole. With a sharp knife, make small incisions all over the bird. Place in a large bowl.

2 Mix the lemon or lime juice with the garlic, ginger, cumin, ground coriander, garam masala, salt and pepper. Rub all over the chicken, working the mixture into the incisions. Cover and leave to marinate in the refrigerator for about 2 hours.

3 Heat the oil in a frying pan, add the onions and fry gently for 8–10 minutes or until soft and golden brown. Add the turmeric and cayenne and fry for a further 2 minutes.

4 Add the yogurt, 15 ml (1 tbsp) at a time. Cook each addition over a high heat, stirring constantly, until the yogurt is absorbed.

5 Transfer the onion and yogurt mixture to a blender or food processor. Add the cashew nuts or almonds and purée until smooth.

6 Place the chicken in a casserole or roasting tin and spread the onion mixture all over the bird. Cover with a lid or foil, then bake in a preheated oven at 180°C (350°F) mark 4 for about 1 hour, basting frequently, until the chicken is tender.

7 Transfer the chicken to a warmed serving dish and spoon over the sauce. Sprinkle with chopped coriander and serve immediately.

CORN-FED CHICKEN SALAD WITH RASPBERRY VINAIGRETTE

Corn-fed chicken has a good flavour. However, if it is unavailable, this salad tastes good made with ordinary chicken breasts.

Serves 4

252 kcals per serving

450 ml (¾ pint) chicken stock
2 bay leaves
1 slice of lemon
few allspice berries
4 skinned corn-fed chicken breast
fillets
mixed salad leaves and herbs
175 g (6 oz) mange-tout, trimmed
225 g (8 oz) seedless green grapes

a few raspberries, to garnish

For the Vinaigrette
225 g (8 oz) raspberries
15 ml (1 tbsp) vegetable oil
10 ml (2 tsp) raspberry vinegar
salt and freshly ground pepper
artificial sweetener, to taste

1 Put the stock, bay leaves, lemon slice and allspice berries in a large deep frying pan. Add the chicken and simmer gently for 10–15 minutes or until tender. Remove from the heat and leave the chicken to cool in the stock.

2 To make the vinaigrette, push the raspberries through a nylon sieve to purée and remove the seeds. Whisk the oil and vinegar into the raspberry purée. Season to taste with salt, pepper and artificial sweetener.

3 When ready to serve, arrange the salad leaves and herbs on four plates. Blanch the mange-tout in boiling water for 1 minute, then drain and rinse under cold running water. Drain again. Arrange the mange-tout on top of the salad leaves with the grapes.

4 Remove the chicken from the stock and drain on absorbent kitchen paper. Slice the chicken thinly and arrange on top of the salad.

5 Whisk the vinaigrette to mix thoroughly, then pour over each salad. Garnish with a few raspberries. Serve the remaining dressing separately.

*T*URKEY SAUTÉ WITH LEMON
AND WALNUTS

The subtle sweetness of this simple-to-make sauté dish gives it a most unusual flavour. Serve with a plain vegetable accompaniment so you can appreciate its flavour to the full.

Serves 4

330 kcals per serving

450 g (1 lb) turkey breast steaks
30 ml (2 tbsp) cornflour
30 ml (2 tbsp) vegetable oil
40 g (1½ oz) walnut halves or pieces
1 green pepper, cored, seeded and
   cut into thin strips

60 ml (4 tbsp) chicken stock
30 ml (2 tbsp) lemon juice
45 ml (3 tbsp) lemon marmalade
5 ml (1 tsp) white wine vinegar
1.25 ml (¼ tsp) soy sauce
salt and freshly ground pepper

1 Cut the turkey flesh into 5 cm (2 inch) pencil-thin strips. Toss in the cornflour.
2 Heat the oil in a large sauté pan, add the walnuts and pepper strips and fry for 2–3 minutes. Remove from the pan with a slotted spoon.
3 Add the turkey strips to the pan and fry in the residual oil for 10 minutes or until golden. Stir in the stock and lemon juice, stirring well to loosen any sediment in the bottom of the pan. Add the lemon marmalade, vinegar, soy sauce and salt and pepper to taste.
4 Return the walnuts and green pepper to the pan. Cook gently for a further 5 minutes or until the turkey is tender. Taste and adjust the seasoning and serve immediately.

Opposite: Fisherman's Pie (page 53)
Overleaf: Stir-fried Chicken with Vegetables and Cashew Nuts (page 61)

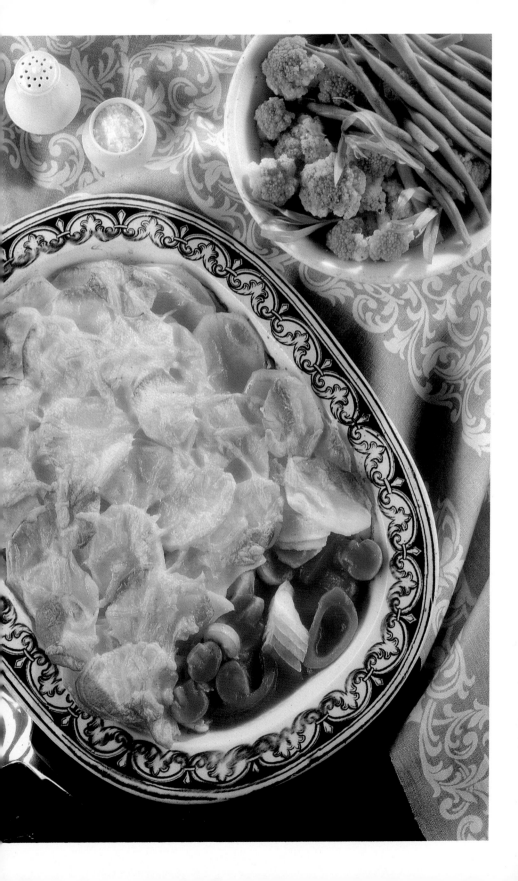

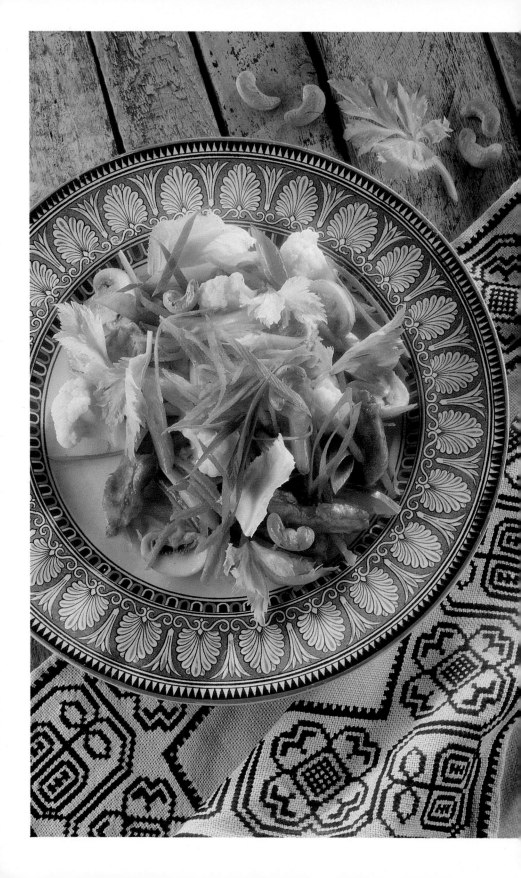

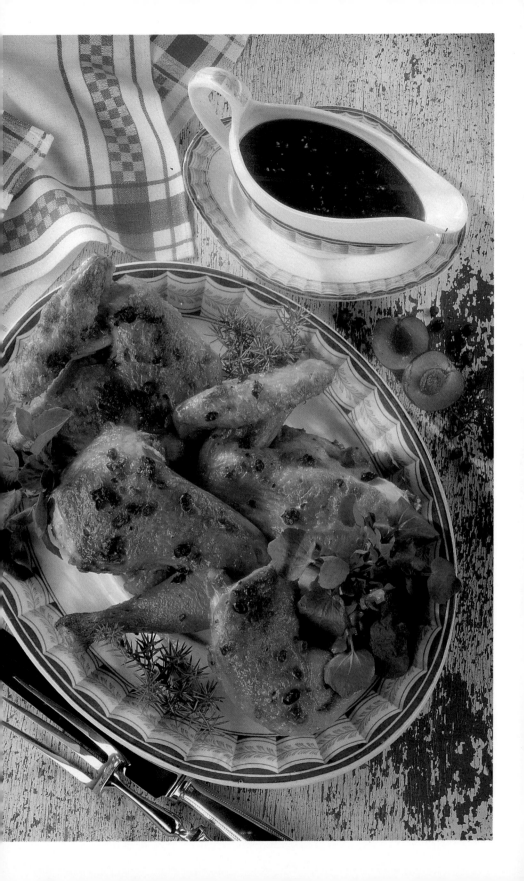

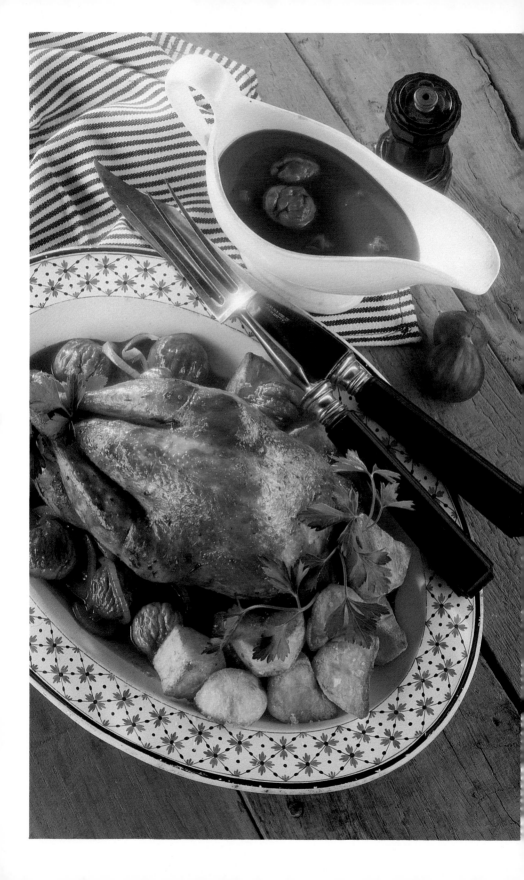

*T*URKEY PAPRIKA WITH PASTA

Quick and easy to make, this meal needs no accompaniment other than a crisp green salad.

Serves 4

301 kcals per serving

15 ml (1 tbsp) vegetable oil
1 medium onion, skinned and sliced
450 g (1 lb) turkey breasts
10 ml (2 tsp) paprika
450 ml (¾ pint) chicken stock
salt and freshly ground pepper

1 green pepper, cored, seeded and
 sliced
100 g (4 oz) small pasta shapes
150 ml (5 fl oz) low-fat natural yogurt
paprika, to garnish

1 Heat the oil in a large sauté pan and fry the onion for 5–10 minutes or until golden brown.
2 Skin the turkey breasts, discard any bone and cut the flesh into small finger-sized pieces.
3 Add the turkey and paprika to the pan and toss over a moderate heat for 2 minutes.
4 Stir in the stock and salt and pepper to taste and bring to the boil. Add the green pepper and pasta, cover and simmer gently for 15–20 minutes or until the turkey and pasta are tender.
5 Stir in the yogurt and adjust the seasoning. To serve, garnish with a little paprika.

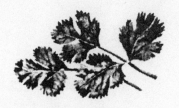

Opposite: Pheasant with Chestnuts (page 70)
Previous page: Grilled Guinea Fowl with Plum and Ginger Sauce (page 69)

*R*ABBIT WITH PRUNES

Surprisingly, rabbit is quite low in fat and, therefore, low in calories. Serve this flavoursome casserole with lightly cooked fresh vegetables.

Serves 4

310 kcals per serving

6-8 back fillets of rabbit, about 450-
    550 g (1-1¼ lb) total weight
15 ml (1 tbsp) whole grain mustard
30 ml (2 tbsp) plain flour
15 ml (1 tbsp) chopped mixed herbs,
    such as basil and parsley
salt and freshly ground pepper

30 ml (2 tbsp) vegetable oil
12 shallots or pickling onions, skinned
3 carrots, scrubbed and sliced
450 ml (¾ pint) chicken stock
5 ml (1 tsp) tomato purée
12 ready-to-eat stoned prunes
fresh herbs, to garnish

1 Brush the rabbit fillets lightly with mustard. Mix together the flour, herbs and salt and pepper to taste. Use to coat the rabbit fillets, reserving the excess flour mixture.

2 Heat the oil in a flameproof casserole. Add the shallots or pickling onions, carrots and rabbit fillets. Cook for about 5 minutes, turning frequently, until the rabbit is sealed. Remove the rabbit and set aside.

3 Stir the reserved flour mixture into the casserole and cook for 1 minute. Add the stock and tomato purée and bring to the boil, stirring. Remove from the heat. Return the rabbit to the casserole and cover.

4 Cook in a preheated oven at 190°C (375°F) mark 5 for 50 minutes. Gently stir in the prunes. Cover again and cook for a further 30 minutes or until the rabbit is tender and cooked through. Garnish with fresh herbs.

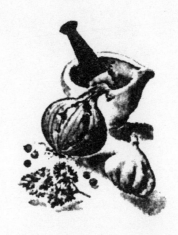

*C*ASSEROLED PIGEONS WITH CIDER AND APPLE

Allow one pigeon per person as the largest weigh only 700 g (1½ lb). Pigeons can be bought frozen. Thaw thoroughly in the refrigerator overnight before cooking.

Serves 4

367 kcals per serving

4 oven-ready pigeons
1 large onion, skinned and sliced into rings
2–3 celery sticks, trimmed and chopped
450 g (1 lb) apples, peeled, cored and thinly sliced
pinch of cayenne

pinch of freshly grated nutmeg
1 bay leaf
salt
600 ml (1 pint) medium or dry cider
few drops of Worcestershire sauce
watercress sprigs and apple slices, to garnish

1 Put the pigeons in a large casserole, either whole or cut in half.

2 Arrange the vegetables and apples around the birds, add the cayenne, nutmeg and bay leaf and season well with salt. Pour over the cider.

3 Cover the casserole and cook in a preheated oven at 150°C (300°F) mark 2 for 2 hours or until the birds are quite tender and the vegetables soft.

4 Remove the birds and the bay leaf with a slotted spoon. Discard the bay leaf and keep the pigeons warm. Purée the cooking liquid and the vegetables in a blender or food processor until smooth.

5 Taste the sauce and if it is too sweet (which will depend on the apples and cider used) add a few drops of Worcestershire sauce.

6 Pour the sauce over the birds and garnish with watercress sprigs and apple slices.

*C*OUSCOUS AND MINT-STUFFED POUSSINS

Serve with raita made from low-fat yogurt, flavoured with mint and chilli powder to taste.

Serves 8

195 kcals per serving

75 g (3 oz) couscous
10 ml (2 tsp) olive oil
6.5 cm (2½ inch) piece of cucumber, finely chopped
3 spring onions, trimmed and finely chopped
15 ml (1 tbsp) chopped fresh mint or 7.5 ml (½ tbsp) dried

15 ml (1 tbsp) lemon juice
salt and freshly ground pepper
4 oven-ready poussins, each weighing about 450 g (1 lb)
mint sprigs and lemon slices, to garnish

1 Place the couscous in a bowl and pour over 150 ml (¼ pint) warm water and the olive oil, then set aside to soak for 10 minutes.
2 Rub the couscous with your fingers to separate the grains. Stir in the cucumber, spring onions, mint, lemon juice and salt and pepper to taste.
3 Spoon the couscous stuffing into the poussins, pressing it in lightly. Twist the wing tips under each bird to hold the neck flaps in place. Tie the legs together with fine string.
4 Place the poussins in a roasting pan, breast-side down, cover with aluminium foil and cook in a preheated oven at 190°C (375°F) mark 5 for 30–45 minutes. Turn the birds over, uncover and continue cooking for a further 10 minutes to brown. The poussins are cooked through when the juices run clear when the thickest part of the leg is pierced with a fine skewer. Serve hot, garnished with mint sprigs and lemon slices.

GRILLED GUINEA FOWL WITH PLUM AND GINGER SAUCE

Nowadays, guinea fowl are bred for the table, so these smallish birds are plumper than the wild guinea fowl. The tender flesh has a delicious flavour rather like gamy chicken, but it must be kept moist during cooking as it has a tendency to dry out.

Serves 4

235 kcals per serving

2 guinea fowl
100 ml (4 fl oz) red wine
1 shallot or 2 spring onions, skinned or trimmed and finely chopped
30 ml (2 tbsp) thick plum or damson jam

1.25–2.5 ml (¼–½ tsp) ground ginger, to taste
salt and freshly ground pepper
25 g (1 oz) butter
30 ml (2 tbsp) crushed juniper berries
watercress sprigs, to garnish

1 Cut each guinea fowl into four joints.

2 Make the plum sauce. Put the wine and shallot or onion in a small saucepan, cover and simmer for 5 minutes or until soft. Add the jam, ginger and salt and pepper to taste. Heat gently until the jam melts, then bring to the boil and simmer for a few minutes or until thickened slightly. Remove from the heat.

3 Melt the butter in a small pan with the juniper berries and salt and pepper to taste. Place the guinea fowl, skin side down, on an oiled grill and brush with half of the juniper berry mixture. Grill under a medium heat for 7 minutes, then turn the guinea fowl over and brush with the remaining mixture. Grill for a further 7 minutes until cooked through and the skin crisp.

4 Just before the guinea fowl are ready to serve, pour the cooking juices into the plum sauce and reheat. Taste and adjust the seasoning. Arrange the guinea fowl portions on a serving platter and garnish with watercress. Serve the sauce separately.

PHEASANT WITH CHESTNUTS

Many supermarkets now sell oven-ready fresh or frozen pheasant during the season, which runs from 1 October to 1 February (10 December in Scotland). You may also be able to buy fresh game from your butcher, in which case ask for the bird to be plucked and drawn.

Serves 4 or 6

620 or 415 kcals per serving

15 ml (1 tbsp) vegetable oil
2 oven-ready pheasants, jointed
2 medium onions, skinned and sliced
225 g (8 oz) peeled chestnuts
45 ml (3 tbsp) plain flour
450 ml (¾ pint) hot chicken stock

150 ml (¼ pint) dry red wine
salt and freshly ground pepper
grated rind and juice of ½ orange
10 ml (2 tsp) redcurrant jelly
1 bouquet garni
chopped fresh parsley, to garnish

1 Heat the oil in a large non-stick frying pan and fry the pheasant joints for about 5 minutes or until browned. Remove from the pan and put into a casserole.
2 Add the onions and chestnuts to the pan and fry in the remaining oil for a few minutes or until brown, then add to the pheasant.
3 Stir the flour into the fat remaining in the pan and cook, stirring, for 2–3 minutes. Remove from the heat and gradually stir in the stock and wine. Bring to the boil, stirring continuously, until thickened and smooth. Season with salt and pepper to taste and pour over the pheasant in the casserole. Add the orange rind and juice, redcurrant jelly and bouquet garni.
4 Cover the casserole and bake in a preheated oven at 180°C (350°F) mark 4 for about 1 hour or until the pheasant is tender. Remove the bouquet garni before serving, garnished with parsley.

*L*EANER MEAT AND OFFAL

WHEN buying meat, look for the new leaner cuts now widely available. Trim off all excess fat before cooking, even when using these cuts. When cooking, it is important to add as little fat as possible, as meat already contains relatively large amounts. Compared with meat, offal is lower in fat, higher in protein and has even more vitamins and minerals.

Grilling and barbecuing are excellent methods of cooking for both meat and offal, since most of the fat can drain away. Meat can also be roasted, if you use no basting fat and stand the joint on a rack inside a roasting tin. Meat is best browned for a pot-roast or casserole by dry-frying in a heavy-based frying pan or casserole dish, or by using just a little low-fat spread, or by brushing the pan with the lightest smear of oil. Always skim the fat from casseroles, stews, gravies and sauces before serving.

Stir-frying is quick, simple and fun and it makes a little meat go a long way. Once you have mastered the basic technique, it's easy to devise your own variations. See our recipe on page 77.

A lot of shop-bought chilled or frozen ready-meals containing meat also contain a lot of fat. Read the labels carefully before buying, or make your own using the low-calorie recipes in this chapter.

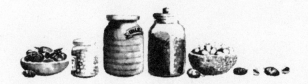

*B*URGUNDY BEEF

Be sure to trim all visible fat from the beef to keep the calorie content of this beef casserole as low as possible.

Serves 4

315 kcals per serving

10 ml (2 tsp) olive oil
550 g (1¼ lb) beef topside, trimmed
  of all fat and cubed
15 g (½ oz) plain flour
30 ml (2 tbsp) brandy
1 onion, skinned and coarsely
  chopped
2 carrots, scrubbed and sliced
1 garlic clove, skinned and crushed
freshly ground pepper

1 bouquet garni
150 ml (¼ pint) red Burgundy
150 ml (¼ pint) hot beef stock
  (optional)
225 g (8 oz) shallots or pickling
  onions, skinned
225 g (8 oz) button mushrooms
lemon juice
chopped fresh parsley, to garnish

1 Brush a heavy-based frying pan with 5 ml (1 tsp) of the oil and heat. Toss the beef in the flour, add to the pan and cook over a medium heat for about 1 minute to seal.

2 Remove the pan from the heat, pour the brandy over and, holding the pan at a safe distance, ignite. When the flame dies down, add the chopped onion, carrots, garlic, pepper to taste and the bouquet garni. Stir for 1 minute, add the wine and heat gradually. When the mixture begins to bubble, pour into an ovenproof casserole with a tight-fitting lid. The meat and vegetables should be covered by the liquid, so add the stock if necessary.

3 Cover and cook in a preheated oven at 150°C (300°F) mark 2 for 1½ hours.

4 Brush the frying pan with the remaining oil, add the shallots or pickling onions and cook over a high heat until browned. Add to the casserole and cook for a further 30 minutes. Add the mushrooms and cook for a further 15 minutes. Add lemon juice to taste. Remove the bouquet garni and serve the casserole while piping hot, garnished with parsley.

MARINATED BEEF AND OLIVE SALAD

This flavoursome beef salad is the perfect main course for an al fresco lunch. Serve with crusty French bread and accompany with chilled Frascati or Soave spritzers.

Serves 4

341 kcals per serving

450 g (1 lb) rolled lean brisket
1 bay leaf
6 peppercorns
1 large bunch of spring onions
12 black olives

450 g (1 lb) French beans
salt and freshly ground pepper
45 ml (3 tbsp) soy sauce
20 ml (4 tsp) lemon juice

1 Put the beef, bay leaf and peppercorns in a saucepan. Add enough water to cover. Bring to the boil, cover and simmer gently for about 1 hour or until the meat is tender. Leave to cool in the cooking liquid for about 2 hours.

2 Trim the spring onions and slice diagonally into thick pieces. Quarter and stone the olives. Trim and halve the French beans. Cook the beans in boiling salted water for 5–10 minutes or until just tender. Drain well, rinse under cold water and drain again thoroughly.

3 Drain the beef and trim off the fat. Slice thinly and cut into 4 cm (1½ inch) long shreds.

4 Put the beef in a bowl and add the spring onions, olives, beans, soy sauce and lemon juice. Toss well together, then season with pepper to taste. (The soy sauce should provide sufficient salt.) Cover and chill in the refrigerator for about 30 minutes before serving.

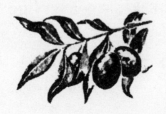

*B*EEF TERIYAKI

Try sake, the Japanese rice wine, in this dish, instead of sherry. Sake is available from larger off-licences. Serve with stir-fried vegetables.

Serves 4

205 kcals per serving

4 beef steaks, such as sirloin, rump or fillet, each weighing about 100 g (4 oz), trimmed of all fat
30 ml (2 tbsp) soy sauce
30 ml (2 tbsp) dry sherry or sake

2.5 ml (½ tsp) finely grated fresh root ginger
1 garlic clove, skinned and crushed
finely sliced spring onions, to garnish

1 Place the steaks in a dish in a single layer. Mix together the soy sauce, dry sherry or sake, ginger and garlic and pour over the steaks. Marinate for at least 30 minutes, turning the steaks occasionally.
2 Cook the steaks under a hot grill for 5–15 minutes, until rare, medium or well done, turning once and basting with the remaining marinade.
3 Place the steaks on a warmed serving platter or individual plates and spoon over any remaining marinade juices. Scatter the sliced spring onions over the top and serve at once.

*G*RILLED LAMB WITH MINT AND LEMON

If fresh mint is unavailable, stir a little mint sauce into the yogurt marinade.

Serves 4

300 kcals per serving

4 shoulder of lamb chops, each weighing about 175 g (6 oz) and about 2 cm (¾ inch) thick, trimmed of all fat
grated rind of 1 lemon
60 ml (4 tbsp) lemon juice, strained

60 ml (4 tbsp) low-fat natural yogurt
1 large garlic clove, skinned and crushed
60 ml (4 tbsp) chopped fresh mint
salt and freshly ground pepper

1 Place the chops in a shallow, non-metallic dish.

2 Mix together the lemon rind, lemon juice, yogurt, garlic, mint and salt and pepper to taste. Spoon over the lamb, cover and refrigerate for at least 12 hours.

3 Place the lamb on a grill rack and spoon over half the marinade.

4 Grill for about 8 minutes on each side, turning the meat once and spooning over the remaining marinade. Serve immediately.

*L*AMB WITH SPINACH

Spicy and rich, this Indian dish of lamb and spinach goes well with plain boiled basmati rice. Serve cucumber raita as a side dish.

Serves 6

355 kcals per serving

900 g (2 lb) boned leg or shoulder of lamb, trimmed of all fat and cubed
90 ml (6 tbsp) low-fat natural yogurt
1 cm (½ inch) piece of fresh root ginger, peeled and chopped
2 garlic cloves, skinned and chopped
2.5 cm (1 inch) cinnamon stick
2 bay leaves
2 green cardamoms
4 black peppercorns

3 whole cloves
5 ml (1 tsp) ground cumin
5 ml (1 tsp) garam masala
1.25–2.5 ml (¼–½ tsp) chilli powder
5 ml (1 tsp) ground coriander
5 ml (1 tsp) salt
450 g (1 lb) fresh or 226 g (8 oz) packet frozen chopped spinach
sprig of mint and lemon slices, to garnish

1 Place the cubes of meat in a bowl. In a separate bowl, mix together the yogurt, ginger, garlic, whole and ground spices and the salt.

2 Spoon the mixture over the meat and mix thoroughly. Cover and leave to marinate at room temperature for about 4 hours.

3 Meanwhile, thoroughly wash and chop the fresh spinach. Thaw the frozen spinach by heating gently in a saucepan.

4 Put the marinated meat in a heavy-based saucepan with the marinade and cook over a low heat for about 1 hour, stirring occasionally, until all the moisture has evaporated and the meat is tender.

5 Stir in the spinach and cook over a low heat for a further 10 minutes. Serve garnished with mint and lemon slices.

PORK TENDERLOIN WITH ORANGE AND GINGER

Pork tenderloin is very lean, as its name suggests, but trim off all visible fat before cooking.

Serves 4 or 6

438 or 292 kcals per serving

grated rind of 1 orange and 1 lemon
50 ml (2 fl oz) orange juice
50 ml (2 fl oz) lemon juice
50 g (2 oz) piece of fresh root ginger, peeled and finely grated or chopped
15 ml (1 tbsp) hoisin sauce
15 ml (1 tbsp) granulated artificial sweetener
1 garlic clove, skinned and crushed

2 pork tenderloins (fillets), about 700 g (1½ lb) total weight, trimmed of all fat
225 g (8 oz) carrots, scrubbed
vegetable oil
300 ml (½ pint) chicken stock
salt and freshly ground pepper
chopped fresh parsley and orange segments, to garnish

1 Stir together the orange and lemon rind and juice. Add the ginger, hoisin sauce, artificial sweetener and garlic.

2 Place the tenderloins in a large, shallow dish. Pour over the ginger mixture and roll the tenderloins to coat completely. Cover and marinate in the refrigerator for at least 3–4 hours – preferably overnight.

3 Cut the carrots into 5 cm (2 inch) matchstick lengths. Drain the pork from the marinade. Lightly grease a large non-stick frying pan with a little oil and heat. Add the pork tenderloins and brown well on all sides. Pour over the ginger marinade and the chicken stock and add the carrots. Cover and simmer very gently for about 15 minutes or until the pork and carrots are cooked through.

4 Remove the tenderloins from the pan with a slotted spoon and slice thickly. Boil the pan juices for 2–3 minutes or until reduced by about half and slightly thickened and syrupy. Adjust the seasoning, adding salt and pepper to taste.

5 Return the tenderloin to the pan, cover and simmer very gently for 1–2 minutes or until heated through. Sprinkle generously with chopped parsley and garnish with orange segments to serve.

STIR-FRIED PORK WITH VEGETABLES

Don't overcook the stir-fry in step 5; soggy beansprouts are most unpleasant and will spoil the dish.

Serves 6

288 kcals per serving

700 g (1½ lb) pork fillet or tenderloin, trimmed of all fat
60 ml (4 tbsp) dry sherry
45 ml (3 tbsp) soy sauce
10 ml (2 tsp) ground ginger
salt and freshly ground pepper
30 ml (2 tbsp) vegetable oil
1–2 garlic cloves, skinned and crushed

225 g (8 oz) courgettes, thickly sliced
30 ml (2 tbsp) cornflour
300 ml (½ pint) cold chicken stock
1 bunch of spring onions, trimmed and finely chopped
175 g (6 oz) beansprouts

1 Cut the pork into thin strips and place in a bowl. Add the sherry, soy sauce, ginger and salt and pepper to taste, then stir well to mix. Set aside.
2 Heat the oil in a wok or large, heavy-based frying pan, add the garlic and fry gently for 1–2 minutes.
3 Add the pork and courgettes to the pan, increase the heat and stir-fry for 2–3 minutes or until lightly coloured, tossing constantly so that the food cooks evenly.
4 Mix the cornflour with the chicken stock and set aside.
5 Add the spring onions and beansprouts to the pork, with the cornflour and stock mixture. Stir-fry until the juices thicken and the ingredients are well combined. Taste and adjust the seasoning, then turn into a warmed serving dish. Serve immediately.

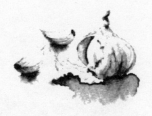

SPICED VEAL WITH PEPPERS

Pie veal is normally sold boned and cubed, which makes it a most convenient cut, but always check the meat before using as some pie veal can be very fatty.

Serves 4

250 kcals per serving

550 g (1¼ lb) pie veal, trimmed of all fat
15 ml (1 tbsp) vegetable oil
2 medium onions, skinned and thinly sliced
2 small red peppers, cored, seeded and thinly sliced
1 garlic clove, skinned and crushed
2.5 ml (½ tsp) ground ginger
2.5 ml (½ tsp) ground turmeric
2.5 ml (½ tsp) ground cumin
2.5 ml (½ tsp) chilli powder
1.25 ml (¼ tsp) ground cloves
225 g (8 oz) tomatoes, skinned and roughly chopped
300 ml (½ pint) low-fat natural yogurt
salt and freshly ground pepper

1   Cut the veal into chunky cubes.
2   Heat the oil in a large saucepan. Add the onions, peppers, garlic and spices and fry for 1 minute. Stir in the chopped tomatoes.
3   Turn the heat to very low and very gradually add the yogurt, stirring well between each addition.
4   Add the veal, with salt and pepper to taste. Cover and simmer gently for 30 minutes.
5   Uncover the pan and cook the veal for a further 30 minutes or until it is tender and the liquid has reduced. Stir occasionally to prevent the meat sticking to the pan. Taste and adjust the seasoning before serving.

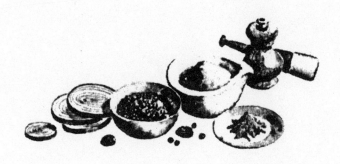

SAUTÉED VEAL WITH COURGETTES AND GRAPEFRUIT

This dish has its own vegetables and therefore needs no accompaniment other than plain boiled pasta, such as tagliatelle.

Serves 4

226 kcals per serving

450 g (1 lb) veal rump or fillet, in one piece, trimmed of all fat
2 grapefruit
30 ml (2 tbsp) olive oil

450 g (1 lb) courgettes, trimmed and thinly sliced
few saffron strands
salt and freshly ground pepper

1   Cut the veal into wafer-thin slices. Place between two sheets of dampened greaseproof paper and bat out with a rolling pin or meat mallet.
2   With a potato peeler, pare the rind from one grapefruit. Cut into thin julienne strips. Squeeze the juice from the grapefruit and reserve.
3   With a serrated knife, peel the remaining grapefruit as you would an apple, removing all skin and pith. Make sure none of the pith remains. Slice the flesh thinly and set aside.
4   Heat half the oil in a large non-stick frying pan. Add a few slices of the veal and sauté for about 2–3 minutes or until well browned on both sides. Transfer to a warmed serving dish, cover and keep warm in the oven while sautéeing the remainder.
5   Heat the remaining oil in the pan, add the courgettes and sauté for 2–3 minutes or until beginning to brown. Add the julienne strips of grapefruit, the saffron strands and 90 ml (6 tbsp) of the reserved grapefruit juice.
6   Bring to the boil, then lower the heat and simmer for 4–5 minutes or until the liquid is well reduced. Stir in the thinly sliced grapefruit and heat through.
7   Add salt and pepper to taste, pour over the veal and serve.

*K*IDNEYS PROVENÇAL

This strongly flavoured dish needs a contrasting bland accompaniment such as plain boiled rice. Follow with a simple green salad and fresh fruit for a complete, well-balanced meal.

Serves 4

211 kcals per serving

12–16 lambs' kidneys
30 ml (2 tbsp) olive oil
1 large onion, skinned and chopped
1–2 garlic cloves, skinned and crushed
3 medium courgettes, trimmed and sliced
4 large tomatoes, skinned and roughly chopped

100 ml (4 fl oz) red wine or stock
10 ml (2 tsp) chopped fresh basil or 5 ml (1 tsp) dried
salt and freshly ground pepper
12 stoned black olives
sprigs of chervil, to garnish

1   Skin the kidneys, then cut each one in half. Snip out the cores with kitchen scissors. Cut each half in two.
2   Heat the oil in a large heavy-based frying pan, add the onion and garlic and fry gently for 5 minutes or until soft but not coloured.
3   Add the kidneys and fry over a low heat for 3 minutes or until they change colour. Shake the pan and toss the kidneys frequently during frying.
4   Add the courgettes, tomatoes and wine or stock and bring to the boil, stirring constantly. Lower the heat and add half the basil with salt and pepper to taste. Simmer gently for 8 minutes or until the kidneys are tender.
5   Add the olives to the pan and heat through for 1–2 minutes. Taste and adjust the seasoning. Sprinkle with the remaining basil and garnish with chervil just before serving. Serve very hot.

*L*IVER WITH CURRIED FRUIT

Plain boiled rice and a little low-fat natural yogurt are healthy accompaniments to this spicy liver dish.

Serves 4

348 kcals per serving

30 ml (2 tbsp) vegetable oil
1 large onion, skinned and thinly sliced
15 ml (1 tbsp) curry powder, or to taste
225 g (8 oz) can pineapple chunks in natural juice, drained, with juice reserved

2 green eating apples, cored and sliced
50 g (2 oz) sultanas
3 large firm tomatoes, quartered
450 g (1 lb) lamb's liver, thinly sliced

1 To prepare the curried fruit, heat half of the oil in a medium saucepan and cook the onion for about 5 minutes or until beginning to soften, then add the curry powder. Stir gently for 1–2 minutes to cook the spices, then add the pineapple juice.
2 Bring to the boil, add the apples and sultanas, cover and cook for about 5 minutes or until the apples are soft.
3 Stir in the pineapple chunks and tomatoes, mixing carefully, and heat through gently.
4 Heat the remaining oil in a large heavy-based frying pan until hot, then quickly cook the liver, a few slices at a time, turning at least once, for about 1 minute on each side.
5 Put the liver on a heated serving plate and keep hot while cooking the remaining slices. Serve with the curried fruit.

PAN-FRIED LIVER WITH TOMATOES

Serve with Chinese egg noodles and a stir-fried vegetable dish of onion, ginger, beansprouts and carrots.

Serves 4

290 kcals per serving

450 g (1 lb) lamb's liver, sliced
30 ml (2 tbsp) Marsala or sweet
  sherry
salt and freshly ground pepper
225 g (8 oz) tomatoes, skinned

30 ml (2 tbsp) vegetable oil
2 medium onions, skinned and finely
  sliced
pinch of ground ginger
150 ml (¼ pint) chicken stock

1 Using a very sharp knife, cut the liver into wafer-thin strips. Place in a shallow bowl with the Marsala or sweet sherry. Sprinkle with freshly ground pepper to taste. Cover and leave to marinate for several hours.

2 Cut the tomatoes into quarters and remove the seeds, reserving the juices. Slice the flesh into fine strips and set aside.

3 Heat the oil in a sauté pan or non-stick frying pan. When very hot, add the liver strips, a few at a time. Shake the pan briskly for about 30 seconds until pearls of blood appear on the liver.

4 Turn the slices and cook for a further 30 seconds only (liver hardens if it is overcooked). Remove from the pan with a slotted spoon and keep warm while cooking the remaining batches.

5 Add the onions and ginger to the residual oil in the pan and cook, uncovered, for about 5 minutes. Add the stock and salt and pepper to taste, return the liver to the pan and add the tomatoes and their juice. Bring just to the boil, then turn into a warmed serving dish and serve immediately.

VARIED VEGETARIAN

MAIN courses without meat, poultry or fish should not be reserved for vegetarians. The recipes in this chapter illustrate just how interesting, varied and colourful main dishes, without a central theme of meat or fish, can be.

Don't make the mistake of thinking that all vegetarian food is low-calorie. Be careful about using lots of fat or oil for softening vegetables. Use a little olive oil for flavour, or a fat-reduced spread. In a vegetarian diet, nuts and cheese are good sources of protein but they are also high in calories and should be used judiciously. Pulses, such as beans, chick-peas and lentils, are protein-packed; make the most of them nutritionally by serving them with grain products such as wholewheat pasta or rice, bulgar wheat, buckwheat, oats or cornmeal.

Dried beans must be soaked overnight before cooking. If you forget, use the quick-soak method. Put the beans into a saucepan and cover with cold water. Bring to the boil, then boil for 10 minutes before removing from the heat. Cover the pan and leave in the same water for 2 hours. Drain and then cook the beans in fresh water for a little longer than the usual time.

Tofu has always been an important ingredient in Chinese cooking and recently it has become much more popular and readily available here. It is made from soya bean curd and provides good, high quality protein, whilst being low in both fat and calories. Unfortunately, it does have rather a 'cranky' image, and lacks flavour. If marinated, however, or cooked in a strongly flavoured sauce, it is a valuable addition to any low-calorie diet. See the recipe for Pepper and Tofu Kebabs on page 93.

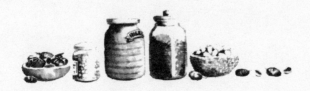

MUSHROOM AND NUT BURGERS WITH FRESH MANGO CHUTNEY

Fresh mango chutney makes an unusual flavoursome accompaniment to these vegetarian burgers.

Serves 4

361 kcals per serving

5 ml (1 tsp) olive oil
1 onion, skinned and finely chopped
100 g (4 oz) mushrooms, coarsely
  chopped
100 g (4 oz) mixed nuts
175 g (6 oz) fresh breadcrumbs
5 ml (1 tsp) yeast extract
10 ml (2 tsp) chopped fresh herbs or
  5 ml (1 tsp) mixed dried herbs

1 egg, size 1
freshly ground pepper

For the Mango Chutney
1 ripe mango
30 ml (2 tbsp) shredded coconut
finely grated rind and juice of 1 lime

1 Lightly grease a baking sheet and set aside. Heat the oil in a heavy-based saucepan. Add the onion, cover and cook over a low heat for 7 minutes or until soft. Add the mushrooms and cook for 3 minutes, then add the nuts and cook for a further 3 minutes.
2 Purée the mixture in a blender or food processor, then transfer to a bowl. Add the remaining ingredients, with pepper to taste, and mix well with a fork.
3 Shape the nut mixture into eight patties, adding a little water if crumbly. Place on the prepared baking sheet and flatten with the palm of the hand. Cook the patties under a preheated medium grill for 4–5 minutes on each side.
4 Meanwhile, make the mango chutney. Peel the mango and cut all the flesh away from the stone. Cut the flesh into small pieces and mix with the remaining ingredients. Serve the burgers hot with the mango chutney.

CARROT AND BUTTER BEAN
SOUFFLÉS

This recipe works best if the carrots are sliced very thinly in a food processor. Serve with a watercress and cucumber salad.

Serves 4

316 kcals per serving

450 g (1 lb) carrots, scrubbed and thinly sliced
salt and freshly ground pepper
25 g (1 oz) low-fat spread
15 ml (1 tbsp) plain flour
425 g (15 oz) can butter beans, drained

75 g (3 oz) Gruyère or Gouda cheese, grated
3 eggs, separated
30 ml (2 tbsp) chopped fresh coriander
10 ml (2 tsp) medium oatmeal or fresh breadcrumbs

1 Cook the carrots in boiling salted water for 10–12 minutes or until well softened. Drain well, reserving 150 ml (¼ pint) of the cooking liquor.
2 Melt the low-fat spread in a saucepan, add the flour and cook, stirring, for 1 minute. Stir in the reserved liquor and bring to the boil, stirring. Simmer for 2 minutes.
3 Place the carrots, sauce, butter beans, cheese and egg yolks in a blender or food processor and purée until smooth. Season with salt and pepper to taste. Turn the mixture into a bowl and fold in the coriander. Whisk the egg whites until stiff and fold in.
4 Spoon the mixture into four well-greased, deep, individual ovenproof dishes. Sprinkle with the oatmeal or breadcrumbs.
5 Bake in a preheated oven at 200°C (400°F) mark 6 for 20–25 minutes or until golden and just firm to the touch.

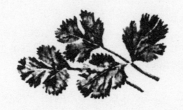

AUBERGINES WITH CANNELLINI BEANS

A hearty filling makes these aubergines a substantial vegetarian meal.

Serves 4

110 kcals per serving

2 medium aubergines
25 g (1 oz) low-fat spread
1 onion, skinned and chopped
1 garlic clove, skinned and crushed
100 g (4 oz) button mushrooms

225 g (8 oz) can cannellini beans,
  drained and rinsed
2 tomatoes, chopped
freshly ground pepper
30 ml (2 tbsp) grated Parmesan cheese

1 Cut the ends off the aubergines and put the aubergines in a large saucepan of boiling water. Cook for 10 minutes or until tender, then drain.
2 Cut the aubergines in half lengthways and scoop out the flesh, leaving a 0.5 cm (¼ inch) shell. Finely chop the flesh and reserve the shells.
3 Melt the low-fat spread in a medium heavy-based saucepan, add the onion, garlic and chopped aubergine flesh and cook gently for 5 minutes.
4 Add the mushrooms, beans, tomatoes and pepper to taste.
5 Stuff the aubergine shells with the prepared mixture and sprinkle with Parmesan cheese. Cook in a preheated oven at 180°C (350°F) mark 4 for 20 minutes or until hot.

SPINACH ROULADE

This is such a low-calorie main dish that you can afford to serve it with a higher-calorie accompaniment such as roast potatoes (see page 97).

Serves 4

177 kcals per serving

900 g (2 lb) fresh spinach, washed
  and trimmed
4 eggs, size 2, separated
salt and freshly ground pepper

100 g (4 oz) low-fat soft cheese with
  garlic and herbs
30 ml (2 tbsp) low-fat natural yogurt

1 Grease and line a 35 x 25 cm (14 x 10 inch) Swiss roll tin. Set aside.
2 Chop the spinach coarsely and place in a saucepan with only the water that clings to the leaves. Cover and simmer for 5 minutes, then drain.

3   Cool the spinach slightly, then beat in the egg yolks and salt and pepper to taste.

4   Whisk the egg whites until stiff, then fold into the spinach mixture until evenly incorporated.

5   Spread the mixture in the prepared Swiss roll tin. Bake in a preheated oven at 200°C (400°F) mark 6 for 20 minutes or until firm. Beat the cheese and yogurt together.

6   When the roulade is cooked, turn it out on to a sheet of greaseproof paper, peel off the lining paper and spread the roulade immediately and quickly with the cheese mixture.

7   Roll up the roulade by gently lifting the greaseproof paper. Place, seam side down, on a serving platter. Serve hot or cold, cut into thick slices.

*M*ARROW STUFFED WITH AUTUMN VEGETABLES

This recipe makes the most of root vegetables. Autumn is the time to make it, when supplies are plentiful. The skin of a good marrow should be shiny and pressing it with the thumb should leave an impression.

Serves 4

88 kcals per serving

550 g (1¼ lb) marrow, peeled and
   halved lengthways
25 g (1 oz) low-fat spread
175 g (6 oz) aubergine, cubed
2 parsnips, peeled and diced
2 carrots, scrubbed and diced
100 g (4 oz) swede, peeled and diced

100 g (4 oz) turnip, peeled and diced
15 ml (1 tbsp) chopped fresh parsley
15 ml (1 tbsp) tomato purée
150 ml (¼ pint) hot vegetable stock
salt and freshly ground pepper
low-fat natural yogurt, to serve

1   Scoop the seeds out of the marrow.

2   Melt the low-fat spread in a large frying pan and lightly fry the vegetables for 10 minutes.

3   Add the parsley, tomato purée and stock. Season with salt and pepper to taste and simmer gently for 15 minutes.

4   Fill one half of the marrow with the mixture. Top with the other half of the marrow and wrap in foil. Bake in a preheated oven at 190°C (375°F) mark 5 for about 45 minutes or until the marrow is tender. Slice and serve at once, accompanied by yogurt.

BUCKWHEAT-STUFFED PEPPERS

The tiny, brown, heart-shaped buckwheat seeds are used in the filling for these peppers. Serve with a mixed leaf salad.

Serves 4

155 kcals per serving

15 ml (1 tbsp) vegetable oil
1 medium onion, skinned and finely chopped
75 g (3 oz) celery, trimmed and chopped
2 garlic cloves, skinned and crushed
75 g (3 oz) buckwheat
50 g (2 oz) mushrooms, finely chopped

300–350 ml (10–12 fl oz) vegetable stock
10 ml (2 tsp) dried oregano
10 ml (2 tsp) chopped fresh parsley
freshly ground pepper
2 tomatoes, chopped
4 peppers, each weighing about 175 g (6 oz)
400 g (14 oz) can tomatoes, drained

1 Heat the oil in a large non-stick frying pan and cook the onion, celery, one garlic clove and the buckwheat for 2 minutes. Add the mushrooms and cook for a further 2 minutes.
2 Add the stock, 7.5 ml (1½ tsp) of the oregano and the chopped parsley. Season with pepper to taste, cover and cook for 15 minutes or until the buckwheat is soft. Mix in the chopped tomatoes.
3 Cut the tops off the peppers and reserve as lids, then cut a thin slice from the base of each one so the peppers stand upright. Core and seed, then blanch the peppers with the lids in a saucepan of boiling water for 5 minutes. Drain well.
4 Fill the peppers with the buckwheat mixture and top with the lids. Stand the peppers in an ovenproof dish and add a little water. Cover and cook in a preheated oven at 180°C (350°F) mark 4 for 30–40 minutes or until cooked through.
5 Purée the canned tomatoes with the remaining garlic and oregano in a blender or food processor. Heat gently and serve with the peppers.

CELERIAC WITH TOMATO SAUCE

Celeriac tastes much like celery, but is a knobbly vegetable that looks like a rough turnip and can vary from about the size of a large apple to as big as a coconut.

Serves 3

160 kcals per serving

1 large onion, skinned and very finely chopped
3 garlic cloves, skinned and crushed
350 g (12 oz) ripe tomatoes, skinned and finely chopped
15 ml (1 tbsp) tomato purée
30 ml (2 tbsp) red wine or red wine vinegar
60 ml (4 tbsp) chopped fresh parsley

5 ml (1 tsp) ground cinnamon
1 bay leaf
salt and freshly ground pepper
2 heads of celeriac, total weight about 900 g (2 lb)
5 ml (1 tsp) lemon juice
50 g (2 oz) fresh breadcrumbs
50 g (2 oz) Cheddar cheese, grated
fresh parsley, to garnish

1 To prepare the tomato sauce, put the onion, garlic and tomatoes in a large heavy-based saucepan and cook gently for about 10 minutes or until very soft.

2 Add the tomato purée, wine, chopped parsley, cinnamon and bay leaf. Season with salt and pepper to taste. Add 450 ml (¾ pint) hot water and bring to the boil, stirring with a wooden spoon to break up the tomatoes.

3 Lower the heat, cover and simmer for 30 minutes, stirring occasionally.

4 Meanwhile, peel the celeriac, then cut into chunky pieces. As you prepare the celeriac, place the pieces in a bowl of water to which the lemon juice has been added, to prevent discoloration.

5 Drain the celeriac, then plunge quickly into a large pan of boiling salted water. Return to the boil and cook for 10 minutes.

6 Drain the celeriac well, then put in an ovenproof serving dish or three individual dishes. Pour over the tomato sauce, discarding the bay leaf, then sprinkle the breadcrumbs and cheese evenly over the top.

7 Bake in a preheated oven at 190°C (375°F) mark 5 for 30 minutes or until the celeriac is tender when pierced with a skewer and the topping is golden brown. Garnish with parsley and serve hot, straight from the dish.

SWEET POTATO LOAF

Buy sweet potatoes which are small and firm; large ones tend to be fibrous.

Makes 12 slices

125 kcals per slice

450 g (1 lb) sweet potatoes
1 carrot, scrubbed and grated
grated rind of 2 oranges
100 g (4 oz) toasted hazelnuts, finely
   chopped
25 g (1 oz) fresh breadcrumbs

450 g (1 lb) ricotta cheese
3 eggs, size 3
15 ml (1 tbsp) black mustard seeds
   (optional)
salt and freshly ground pepper
watercress, to garnish

1   Grease a 900 g (2 lb) loaf tin and line with lightly greased greaseproof paper. Set aside.
2   Wrap the potatoes in foil and bake in a preheated oven at 180°C (350°F) mark 4 for about 1 hour or until soft. Increase the oven temperature to 200°C (400°F) mark 6. Unwrap the potatoes, cool slightly, peel and mash. Add the carrot, orange rind, hazelnuts and breadcrumbs.
3   Blend the ricotta cheese and eggs in a blender or food processor until smooth. Add to the potato mixture and mix well.
4   Heat the mustard seeds, if using, in a frying pan until the seeds pop. Add to the bowl, mix well and season with salt and pepper to taste.
5   Spoon the mixture into the prepared tin and cover with foil. Place in a roasting pan and pour in enough hot water to come halfway up the sides of the loaf tin.
6   Cook in a preheated oven at 200°C (400°F) mark 6 for 1 hour. Remove the foil and cook for a further 15 minutes. Remove from the oven and leave to stand for 5 minutes before turning out.

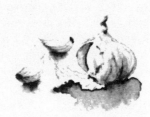

*R*ED KIDNEY BEAN GOULASH WITH OAT AND HERB DUMPLINGS

The dumplings add extra substance to this vegetable stew, without adding too many calories.

Serves 4

204 kcals per serving

225 g (8 oz) dried red kidney beans, soaked for 8–12 hours
25 g (1 oz) low-fat spread
2 onions, skinned and chopped
2 celery sticks, trimmed and chopped
100 g (4 oz) mushrooms, sliced
1 green pepper, cored, seeded and sliced
15 ml (1 tbsp) paprika

400 g (14 oz) can chopped tomatoes

For the Oat and Herb Dumplings
100 g (4 oz) rolled oats
50 g (2 oz) breadcrumbs
15 ml (1 tbsp) chopped fresh herbs
salt and freshly ground pepper
50 g (2 oz) polyunsaturated margarine

1 Drain the beans, put them in a saucepan and cover with water. Boil for 10–15 minutes, skim the surface, then lower the heat, cover and simmer for 35–45 minutes or until just tender. Drain.
2 In a flameproof casserole, melt the low-fat spread and cook the onion and celery for 3 minutes. Add the mushrooms and pepper and cook for 2 minutes.
3 Stir in the paprika, then add the tomatoes with their juice and 450 ml (³/₄ pint) water. Bring to the boil, stirring. Add the beans, lower the heat, cover and simmer for 30 minutes, stirring occasionally.
4 Meanwhile, make the dumplings. Place the oats and breadcrumbs in a bowl and stir in the herbs and salt and pepper to taste. Rub in the margarine until well mixed. Stir in 30 ml (2 tbsp) cold water and mix to a dough. Divide into eight pieces and roll into balls.
5 Float the dumplings on the top of the goulash. Cover and simmer gently for 20 minutes. Serve hot.

VEGETABLE COUSCOUS

This vegetarian dish is a complete meal in itself. Couscous is now readily available from supermarkets.

Serves 4

375 kcals per serving

100 g (4 oz) chick-peas, soaked for 8–12 hours
225 g (8 oz) couscous
15 ml (1 tbsp) vegetable oil
2 onions, skinned and chopped
1 garlic clove, skinned and crushed
5 ml (1 tsp) ground cumin
5 ml (1 tsp) ground coriander

1.25 ml (¼ tsp) chilli powder
2 leeks, trimmed and sliced
2 carrots, scrubbed and sliced
600 ml (1 pint) vegetable stock
3 courgettes, trimmed and sliced
1 large tomato, coarsely chopped
50 g (2 oz) raisins

1 Drain the chick-peas, put in a saucepan, cover with water and boil for 10–15 minutes. Lower the heat and simmer for 40–50 minutes or until just tender, then drain.

2 Meanwhile, put the couscous in a bowl and add 450 ml (¾ pint) cold water. Leave to soak for 10–15 minutes or until the water is absorbed.

3 Heat the oil in a large saucepan, add the onion and cook for 5 minutes. Add the garlic and spices and cook, stirring, for 1 minute. Add the leeks, carrots and stock. Bring to the boil.

4 Line a large sieve with muslin or all-purpose kitchen cloth and place over the vegetable stew. Put the couscous in the sieve. Cover the whole pan with foil to enclose the steam and simmer for 20 minutes.

5 Add the chick-peas, courgettes, tomato and raisins to the stew. Replace the sieve and fluff up the couscous with a fork. Cover and simmer for 10 minutes. Spread the couscous in a large serving dish and spoon the vegetable stew on top.

*P*EPPER AND TOFU KEBABS

Tofu is a very low-fat source of protein. In this recipe, it is first marinated in a spicy yogurt mixture, then grilled.

Serves 4

205 kcals per serving

450 g (1 lb) tofu, cut into 2.5 cm
  (1 inch) cubes
1 large red pepper, cored, seeded
  and cut into squares
1 large green pepper, cored, seeded
  and cut into squares
grated rind and juice of 2 limes or
  1 lemon
45 ml (3 tbsp) olive oil
salt and freshly ground pepper

30 ml (2 tbsp) low-fat natural yogurt
30 ml (2 tbsp) soy sauce
1 garlic clove, skinned and finely
  chopped
1.25 ml ($^1/_4$ tsp) ground cumin
1.25 ml ($^1/_4$ tsp) curry powder
8 cherry tomatoes or 4 tomatoes, cut
  into wedges
shredded lettuce, to serve

1   Put the tofu and pepper pieces in a shallow dish. Mix together the lime or lemon rind and juice, olive oil, salt and pepper to taste, yogurt, soy sauce, garlic and spices. Spoon evenly over the tofu and peppers. Cover and chill for 3–4 hours, turning the tofu and peppers occasionally.

2   Remove the tofu and pepper cubes from the marinade and thread on to skewers, alternating with the tomatoes. Cook under a preheated grill for 3–4 minutes, then turn, brush with the marinade and cook for a further 3–4 minutes. Serve on a bed of shredded lettuce.

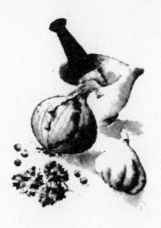

*G*ADO GADO

This traditional Indonesian salad is made of a mixture of cooked and raw vegetables which may be varied according to seasonal availability. It is served with a spicy peanut sauce.

Serves 4

260 kcals per serving

100 g (4 oz) French beans, topped and tailed

225 g (8 oz) white cabbage, finely shredded

100 g (4 oz) carrots, scrubbed and cut into matchsticks

100 g (4 oz) fresh beansprouts

5 cm (2 inch) piece of cucumber, sliced

4 eggs, hard-boiled and sliced

For the Peanut Sauce

50 g (2 oz) desiccated coconut

15 ml (1 tbsp) vegetable or groundnut (peanut) oil

1 small onion, skinned and chopped

75 g (3 oz) natural crunchy peanut butter

5 ml (1 tsp) hot chilli powder

5 ml (1 tsp) sugar

15 ml (1 tbsp) lime juice

1 Bring a saucepan of water to the boil, add the beans and cook for 2 minutes. Add the cabbage and cook for a further 1 minute. Drain, then rinse under cold running water until completely cold. Drain well.

2 Put the blanched vegetables in a large shallow bowl with the carrots and beansprouts and mix well. Arrange the cucumber and egg slices alternately over the vegetables. Chill while preparing the sauce.

3 To make the peanut sauce, place the coconut in a bowl and pour over 300 ml (½ pint) boiling water. Leave to infuse for 20 minutes, then strain through a sieve over a bowl, using a wooden spoon to press out as much liquid as possible. Reserve the liquid and discard the coconut.

4 Heat the oil in a saucepan, add the onion and cook for about 5 minutes or until softened. Add the peanut butter, chilli powder and sugar and mix well. Stir in the strained coconut liquid and bring to the boil. Simmer for 5 minutes or until the sauce has thickened. Remove from the heat, stir in the lime juice and leave to cool. Serve the salad with some of the sauce poured over and the remainder served separately.

CRISP VEGETABLES AND SALADS

WHEN following a calorie-restricted diet, vegetable accompaniments so often get forgotten and yet they can be an exciting part of any main course. Steamed or carefully boiled vegetables are the best option if you are eating a high-calorie main dish. Always add vegetables (even roots) to a small amount of boiling water, to maximize vitamin retention. Toss steamed or boiled vegetables in chopped fresh herbs and freshly ground black pepper or coriander for extra flavour. Purée potatoes, carrots, parsnips and swede with semi-skimmed milk instead of butter, and flavour with freshly grated nutmeg, ground mixed spice or cinnamon. For more inspiration, turn to the recipes in this chapter to fire your imagination and turn your vegetables into dishes to be savoured in their own right. These are all perfect for livening up an otherwise dull fillet of chicken or fish, a plain omelette or a grilled chop.

Most of the salads in this chapter could also make a refreshing meal for a summer lunch or supper, if served with wholemeal bread spread sparingly with low-fat soft cheese. If you are a pudding lover, there's nothing wrong with having the occasional meal consisting of one of these very low-calorie salads, followed by a slightly larger helping of one of the delicious desserts on page 105, as long as you don't do it too often (and your daily calorie intake remains roughly on target)!

Finally, we've included a low-calorie yogurt dressing for you to serve with your own salad and vegetable recipes.

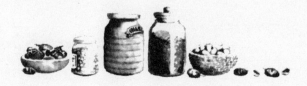

CREAMED GARLIC POTATOES

This comparatively high-calorie vegetable accompaniment is best served with plain grilled fish or meat.

Serves 6

207 kcals per serving

1.4 kg (3 lb) old potatoes, peeled and
    roughly chopped
salt and freshly ground pepper

1 garlic clove, skinned and crushed
45 ml (3 tbsp) Greek yogurt
grated nutmeg, to serve

1   Cook the potatoes in boiling salted water for 15–20 minutes or until very tender. Drain well, then sieve or press through a potato ricer until very smooth. Return to the saucepan.
2   Beat in the garlic and yogurt. Adjust the seasoning and reheat gently before serving sprinkled with grated nutmeg.

ROSTI

Try this nutritious version of the traditional Swiss fried potato dish, made with grated potato.

Serves 4

130 kcals per serving

450 g (1 lb) potatoes, scrubbed and
    grated
1 onion, skinned and grated
45 ml (3 tbsp) chopped fresh parsley

1.25 ml (¼ tsp) grated nutmeg
salt and freshly ground pepper
15 ml (1 tbsp) vegetable oil
parsley sprig, to garnish

Opposite: Burgundy Beef (page 72)
Overleaf: Vegetable Couscous (page 92)

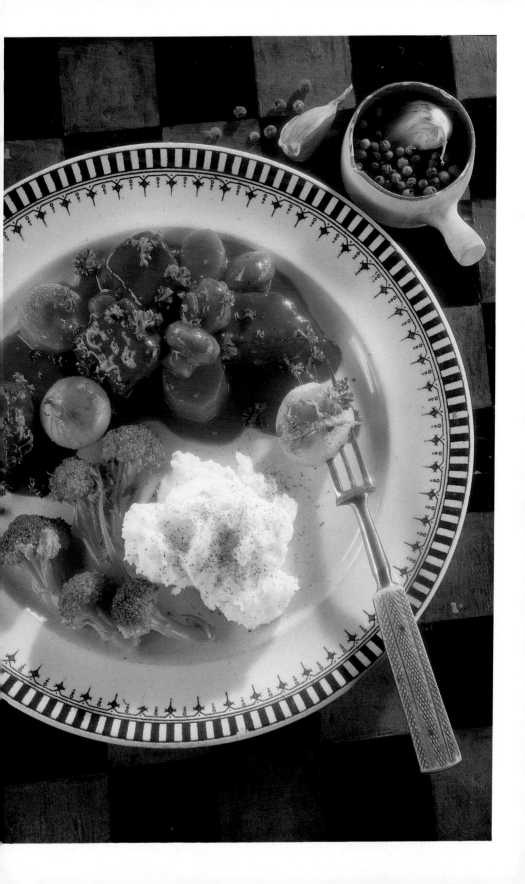

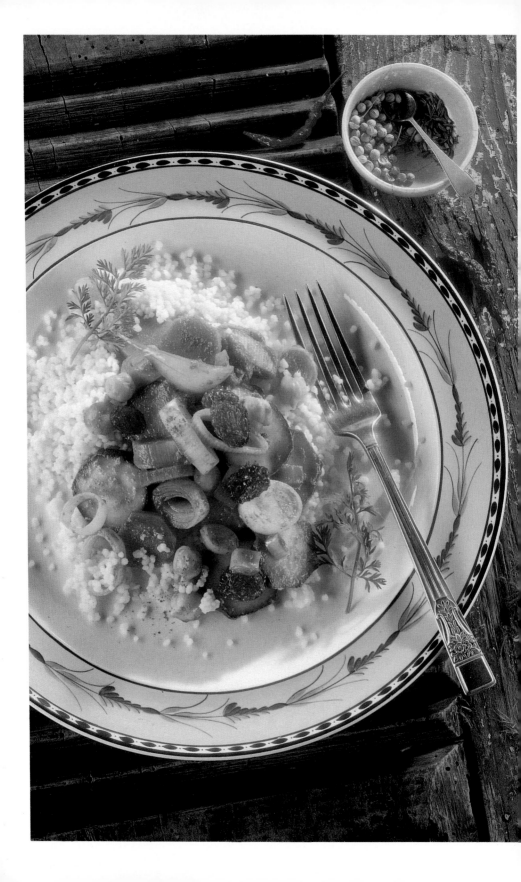

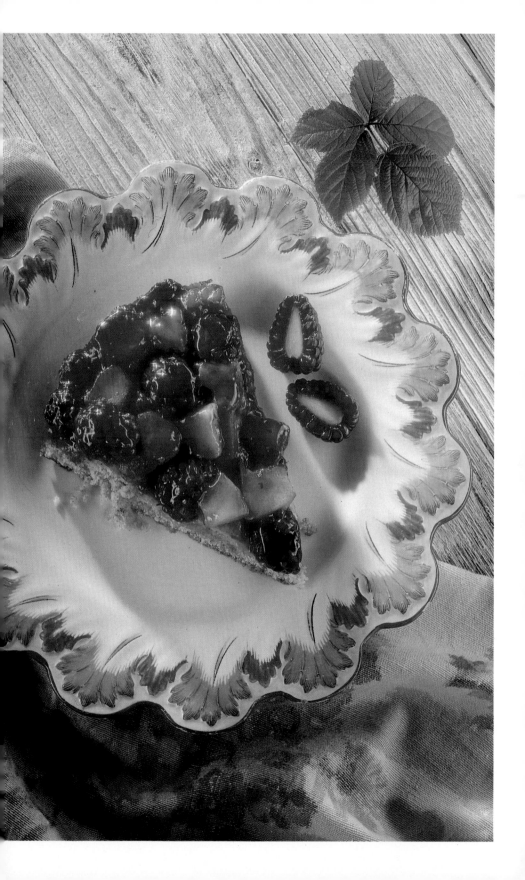

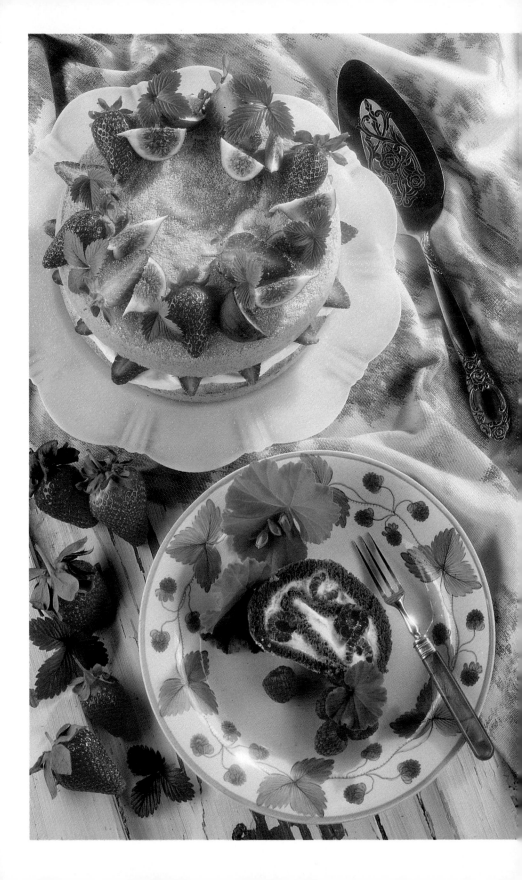

1 Thoroughly mix together the potatoes, onion, parsley, nutmeg and salt and pepper to taste.

2 Heat the oil in a large non-stick frying pan and add the potato mixture, patting it down to form a firm cake. Cook very gently for about 15 minutes on each side, until firm and golden. If the Rosti breaks up a bit when you turn it, don't worry, as it is easy to pat back into shape with a spoon.

3 Remove the Rosti from the pan and serve immediately, garnished with a sprig of parsley.

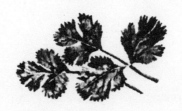

*R*OAST POTATOES

Although lower in calories than usual, this is still a high-calorie accompaniment so is best served with plain grilled fish or chicken dishes.

Serves 4 or 6

186 or 124 kcals per serving

700 g (1½ lb) old potatoes, peeled   salt
15 ml (1 tbsp) vegetable oil   chopped fresh parsley

1 Cut the potatoes into 2.5 cm (1 inch) chunks.

2 Put the oil in a large, shallow non-stick roasting pan and heat in a pre-heated oven at 220°C (425°F) mark 7 until very hot.

3 Add the potato pieces to the oil and shake well so that all sides are coated. Bake in the oven for 1 hour, turning occasionally, until the potatoes are really crisp and golden brown. Sprinkle with a little salt and parsley before serving.

Opposite: Red Fruit Gâteau (page 115); Chocolate and Crushed Raspberry Roulade (page 107)
Previous page: Apple and Blackberry Upside-down Pudding (page 106)

GLAZED CARROT RIBBONS WITH LEMON AND GARLIC

Quick and easy to prepare, this is good served with any fish recipe. It's important only just to cover the carrots with water as you want the liquid to evaporate before they become soft and mushy.

Serves 4

65 kcals per serving

450 g (1 lb) carrots, scrubbed
pared rind of 1 lemon
25 g (1 oz) low-fat spread
15 ml (1 tbsp) sugar

1 garlic clove, skinned and crushed
salt and freshly ground pepper
chopped fresh parsley, to garnish

1 Cut the carrots on the slant into thin slices. Place in a small saucepan with the lemon rind, low-fat spread, sugar, garlic and salt and pepper to taste. Just cover with cold water.
2 Bring to the boil, then cook over a moderate to high heat for about 12 minutes or until the carrots are tender and all the liquid has evaporated. Shake the pan to prevent the carrots sticking.
3 Serve garnished with parsley.

SPRING GREENS AND MUSHROOMS

Steaming the spring greens retains both their vitamins and their crunchiness. The mushrooms are cooked only briefly in lime or lemon juice, so this whole dish has a fairly crisp texture.

Serves 4

25 kcals per serving

225 g (8 oz) spring greens, stalks
   discarded
100 g (4 oz) mushrooms, sliced

juice of 1 lime or ½ lemon
freshly ground pepper
15 ml (1 tbsp) sunflower seeds

1 Finely shred the spring greens and place in a steamer, sieve or colander over a saucepan of gently boiling water. Cover and steam for 6–8 minutes or until the greens are almost cooked but still crunchy.

2 Meanwhile, put the mushrooms, lime or lemon juice and 30 ml (2 tbsp) water in a large saucepan and cook for 3 minutes. Drain off all but 15 ml (1 tbsp) of the liquid, then add the spring greens to the pan. Season with pepper to taste and cook over a high heat for 2 minutes.

3 Place in a warmed serving dish, scatter the sunflower seeds over and serve hot.

*C*OURGETTES IN ORANGE SAUCE

Use a light soy sauce for this recipe; it has a more delicate flavour than the dark version.

Serves 4

65 kcals per serving

350 g (12 oz) courgettes, trimmed,
  halved lengthways and cut into
  10 cm (4 inch) lengths
4 spring onions, trimmed and finely
  chopped
5 ml (1 tsp) grated fresh root ginger
45 ml (3 tbsp) cider vinegar
15 ml (1 tbsp) soy sauce

10 ml (2 tsp) sugar
30 ml (2 tbsp) dry sherry
45 ml (3 tbsp) vegetable stock
finely grated rind and juice of
  1 orange
7.5 ml (1½ tsp) cornflour
1 orange, peeled and segmented

1 Cook the courgettes in boiling water for 3–5 minutes or until just tender.

2 Meanwhile, put the remaining ingredients, except the cornflour and orange segments, into a saucepan and bring to the boil. Lower the heat and simmer gently for 4 minutes.

3 Mix the cornflour with a little water to make a smooth paste, then stir into the sauce and cook for 2 minutes, stirring continuously, until the sauce thickens.

4 Drain the courgettes and return them to the pan. Pour over the sauce and add the orange segments. Heat through briefly before serving.

NORMANDY BEANS

To make the apple purée, slit a small eating apple around the middle and bake in an ovenproof dish at 200°C (400°F) mark 6 for 45 minutes. Alternatively, cook in a microwave cooker on MEDIUM for 5 minutes. Set aside to cool, then remove and discard the skin and core. Purée in a blender or food processor or mash by hand.

Serves 4

50 kcals per serving

350 g (12 oz) French beans, trimmed and cut into 2.5 cm (1 inch) pieces
1 spring onion, trimmed and chopped
45 ml (3 tbsp) unsweetened apple purée (see above)

15 ml (1 tbsp) low-calorie vinaigrette
5 ml (1 tsp) chopped fresh parsley
25 g (1 oz) flaked almonds, toasted
salt and freshly ground pepper

1 Cook the beans in boiling water for about 5 minutes or until tender but still crunchy. Drain, then return to the pan.
2 Add the spring onion, apple purée and vinaigrette. Toss over a high heat for about 1 minute, then cover and cook over a gentle heat for 2–3 minutes, stirring occasionally. Add the parsley, almonds and salt and pepper to taste before serving.

HOT BEETROOT WITH DILL

Leaving the peel on the beetroot during cooking preserves the vitamins.

Serves 4 or 6

75–50 kcals per serving

550 g (1¼ lb) raw beetroot, trimmed
15 ml (1 tbsp) chopped fresh dill or 10 ml (2 tsp) dried dill weed
30 ml (2 tbsp) lemon juice

75 ml (3 fl oz) low-fat natural yogurt
50 ml (2 fl oz) soured cream
salt and freshly ground pepper

1 Place the whole beetroot in a saucepan of boiling water and simmer for about 45 minutes or until just tender. Drain and leave until cool enough to handle.

2 Peel the beetroot, then cut into thin slices. Arrange in a dish and keep warm.

3 Mix the dill with the lemon juice, then stir in the yogurt and soured cream. Season with salt and pepper to taste. Spoon the dressing over the beetroot and serve at once.

COURGETTE AND TOASTED PINENUT SALAD

Do not add the apples to this salad until just before serving, to prevent discoloration.

Serves 8

99 kcals per serving

450 g (1 lb) courgettes, trimmed and thinly sliced
½ head of endive (see page 103)
2 oranges
60 ml (4 tbsp) low-calorie vinaigrette

15 ml (1 tbsp) chopped fresh parsley (optional)
salt and freshly ground pepper
30 ml (2 tbsp) toasted pinenuts or slivered, blanched almonds
2 tart green eating apples

1 Blanch the courgettes in boiling water for 1 minute. Drain and refresh under cold running water. Leave to cool completely, then pat dry with absorbent kitchen paper. Cover and refrigerate. Wash the endive, dry and place in a polythene bag. Chill in the refrigerator.

2 With a serrated knife and holding the fruit over a bowl to catch the juice, cut all the peel and pith away from the oranges. Cut down between the membranes to release the segments into the bowl.

3 Whisk together the dressing, parsley, if using, and salt and pepper to taste. Add to the orange segments with the pinenuts or almonds.

4 Just before serving, halve, core and thinly slice the apples into the dressing mixture. Add the courgettes and endive. Stir well. Adjust the seasoning and serve immediately.

FRESH SPINACH AND BABY CORN SALAD

If fresh baby sweetcorn are not available, look for the pre-cooked canned variety.

Serves 8

81 kcals per serving

350 g (12 oz) fresh young spinach
175 g (6 oz) fresh baby sweetcorn
50 ml (2 fl oz) olive oil
1 garlic clove, skinned and crushed
15 ml (1 tbsp) white wine vinegar
10 ml (2 tsp) Dijon mustard

5 ml (1 tsp) caster sugar
salt and freshly ground pepper
100 g (4 oz) alfalfa sprouts
1 head of chicory, trimmed and
  shredded

1 Wash the spinach well in several changes of cold water. Remove any coarse stalks. Drain well and pat dry on absorbent kitchen paper. Refrigerate in a polythene bag until required.
2 Halve the sweetcorn cobs lengthways. Cook in boiling water for about 10 minutes or until just tender. Drain and refresh under cold running water. Cover and refrigerate.
3 Whisk together the olive oil, garlic, vinegar, mustard and sugar. Season with salt and pepper to taste.
4 Mix together the spinach, sweetcorn, alfalfa sprouts and chicory, toss in the dressing and serve immediately.

STRAWBERRY AND CUCUMBER SALAD

This attractive and refreshing fruit and vegetable combination is the perfect summertime accompaniment to cold meats.

Serves 4

40 kcals per serving

1 small cucumber
10 ml (2 tsp) chopped fresh
  mint
freshly ground pepper

200 ml (7 fl oz) unsweetened apple
  juice
225 g (8 oz) strawberries, hulled
mint sprigs, to garnish

1 With the prongs of a fork, scrape down the sides of the cucumber to make a ridged effect. Slice the cucumber very thinly and lay in a shallow dish. Sprinkle with the chopped mint and pepper to taste. Pour 150 ml (¼ pint) of the apple juice over and chill in the refrigerator for 15 minutes.
2 Slice the strawberries if large; otherwise, cut them in half. Put into a small bowl and pour the remaining apple juice over. Chill for 15 minutes.
3 Drain the cucumber and strawberries and arrange them attractively on a serving dish. Garnish with mint sprigs.

*E*NDIVE, ORANGE AND HAZELNUT SALAD

Endive is rather like a lettuce with very crinkly leaves, ranging through shades of green and yellow. It is sometimes sold as 'frisée'. Endive wilts quickly, so buy it fresh when needed and don't store for more than a day.

Serves 4 or 6

94 or 63 kcals per serving

4 large oranges
1 head of endive, torn into small
  pieces
1 bunch of watercress, trimmed and
  torn into sprigs

1 small red pepper, cored, seeded
  and cut into thin strips
150 ml (5 fl oz) low-fat natural yogurt
salt and freshly ground pepper
25 g (1 oz) hazelnuts

1 Using a serrated knife, cut all the peel and pith away from three of the oranges. Cut down between the membranes to release the segments. Mix the orange segments with the endive, watercress and pepper in a large salad bowl.
2 To make the dressing, finely grate the rind from the remaining orange into a small bowl, then squeeze in the juice. Whisk in the yogurt and season to taste with salt and pepper.
3 Spread the hazelnuts on a baking sheet and toast lightly under a hot grill. Turn the nuts on to a clean tea-towel and rub off the loose skins. Roughly chop the nuts.
4 Just before serving, drizzle the dressing over the salad and sprinkle with the nuts. Serve at once while the nuts are still crunchy.

GREEK SALAD

Serve this salad with grilled or barbecued fish, or as a meal on its own.

Serves 8

120 kcals per serving

900 g (2 lb) ripe tomatoes, sliced
225 g (8 oz) cucumber
225 g (8 oz) feta cheese
100 g (4 oz) stoned black olives
2 large green peppers, cored, seeded
and cut into strips

5 ml (1 tsp) dried oregano
30 ml (2 tbsp) olive oil
30 ml (2 tbsp) low-calorie vinaigrette
freshly ground black pepper

1 Place the tomatoes in a shallow serving dish.
2 Split the cucumber into two long strips, then slice thickly. Cut the feta cheese into 2 cm (¾ inch) cubes.
3 To serve, scatter the olives, cucumber, cheese and green pepper over the tomatoes. Sprinkle with oregano, oil and vinaigrette and season to taste.

YOGURT DRESSING

A useful recipe for a low-fat dressing, suitable for serving with most salads or as a substitute for butter with baked potatoes.

Makes 150 ml (¼ pint)

10 kcals per 15 ml (1 tbsp)

150 ml (5 fl oz) low-fat natural yogurt
10 ml (2 tsp) white wine vinegar
5 ml (1 tsp) clear honey

10 ml (2 tsp) chopped fresh mint
salt and freshly ground pepper

In a small bowl, mix together the yogurt, vinegar, honey and mint with a fork. Season with salt and pepper to taste.

VARIATIONS
1 Omit the mint and add 1 small garlic clove, skinned and crushed.
2 Add other chopped fresh herbs in season or chopped chillies or curry paste, to taste.

DELICIOUS DESSERTS

WHEN you think about low-calorie meals they probably exclude desserts. The sweet things in life, especially desserts, are usually forbidden to those who are watching their weight. Fresh fruit, yogurt and low-fat cheese are all good, healthy, calorie-conscious endings to a meal, but, let's be honest, meal times can get a bit tedious if limited to these, especially if you have a sweet tooth.

In this chapter we show you how to make some lower-calorie desserts that are delicious and tempting enough to appeal to dieters and non-dieters alike. We've even included a chocolate roulade!

If making your own favourite desserts, try to follow the principles laid down here – don't add lots of sugar to fruit-based pies and puddings, let the natural fruit flavour come through. If you can't educate your palate to save calories, try sweetening with a little artificial sweetener instead. Use thick creamy Greek yogurt or fromage frais in place of double cream or try one of the new fat-reduced double cream substitutes.

Likewise, avoid serving puddings with lashings of cream, custard or ice cream. Make custard with semi-skimmed milk and sweeten very lightly; serve low-fat yogurt, Greek yogurt or a fat-reduced cream substitute as an accompaniment if necessary (not forgetting to include them in your calorie calculations); or make a refreshing fruit sauce from lightly poached fruits, puréed and sweetened with a little artificial sweetener.

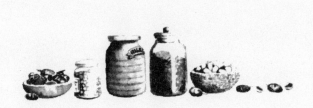

*A*PPLE AND BLACKBERRY
UPSIDE-DOWN PUDDING

A moist sponge topped with a layer of tart blackberries and apples. Best served warm.

Serves 8

190 kcals per serving

For the Topping
90 ml (6 tbsp) reduced-sugar
    raspberry jam
350 g (12 oz) blackberries
1 large eating apple, peeled, cored
    and roughly chopped

For the Cake
75 g (3 oz) self-raising flour
75 g (3 oz) self-raising wholemeal
    flour

5 ml (1 tsp) baking powder
large pinch of salt
1 egg
finely grated rind and juice of 1 large
    orange
30 ml (2 tbsp) semi-skimmed milk
75 g (3 oz) low-fat spread
75 g (3 oz) caster sugar

1 Grease a 23 cm (9 inch) round spring-release cake tin.
2 To make the topping, gently heat the jam in a small saucepan and pour into the prepared cake tin. Arrange the blackberries and apple evenly over the base of the cake tin.
3 To make the cake, put all the ingredients into a large bowl and beat until smooth and glossy. Carefully spread over the fruit and level the surface.
4 Bake in a preheated oven at 190°C (375°F) mark 5 for about 1 hour or until well risen and firm to the touch. Cover the top with a double sheet of greaseproof paper after 40 minutes to prevent overbrowning.
5 Leave the pudding to cool in the tin for 5 minutes, then turn out on to a serving plate.

*C*HOCOLATE AND CRUSHED
RASPBERRY ROULADE

Do not worry if the roulade cracks as you roll it; the cracks are part of its charm.

Serves 8

137 kcals per serving

For the Roulade
50 g (2 oz) plain chocolate
30 ml (2 tbsp) cocoa powder
30 ml (2 tbsp) semi-skimmed
 milk
3 eggs, separated
75 g (3 oz) plus 10 ml (2 tsp) caster
 sugar

For the Filling
175 g (6 oz) natural fromage frais
225 g (8 oz) raspberries

For the Decoration
5 ml (1 tsp) icing sugar
few raspberries
geranium or mint leaves

1 Grease a 23×33 cm (9×13 inch) Swiss roll tin, line with greaseproof paper and grease the paper.
2 To make the roulade, break the chocolate into small pieces. Place in a heatproof bowl standing over a pan of simmering water and heat gently until the chocolate has melted. Stir in the cocoa powder and milk.
3 Whisk the egg yolks and 75 g (3 oz) sugar together in a bowl until very thick and pale in colour. Beat in the chocolate mixture. Whisk the egg whites until stiff, then fold carefully into the mixture. Pour into the prepared tin and spread out evenly.
4 Bake in a preheated oven at 180°C (350°F) mark 4 for 20–25 minutes or until well risen and firm to the touch.
5 While the roulade is cooking, lay a piece of greaseproof paper on a flat work surface and sprinkle with the remaining caster sugar. When the roulade is cooked, turn it out on to the paper. Carefully peel off the lining paper. Cover the roulade with a warm, damp tea-towel and leave to cool.
6 To make the filling, spread the fromage frais over the roulade. Sprinkle with the raspberries, then crush them slightly with a fork. Starting from one of the narrow ends, carefully roll up the roulade, using the greaseproof paper to help. Transfer the roulade to a serving plate and dust with the icing sugar. Decorate with raspberries and geranium or mint leaves.

*O*RANGE SEMOLINA SOUFFLÉS

These individual soufflés, baked in orange peel shells, are good served with thinly sliced oranges sprinkled with a little orange-flavoured liqueur or orange flower water.

Serves 6

110 kcals per serving

5 large juicy oranges
25 g (1 oz) granulated sugar
25 g (1 oz) semolina

3 eggs, separated
a little icing sugar, for dusting

1 Finely grate the rind from two of the oranges. Squeeze the juice from as many of the oranges as needed to make 300 ml (½ pint) juice.
2 Halve the remaining oranges and scoop out the flesh. Eat separately or use in another recipe. You need six clean orange halves to serve the soufflés in. Cut a thin slice from the bottom of each so that they stand flat.
3 Place the orange juice and rind, sugar and semolina in a small saucepan and simmer until thickened, stirring all the time.
4 Cool slightly, then stir in the egg yolks. Whisk the egg whites until stiff and fold into the mixture. Spoon into the reserved orange peel shells and stand on a baking sheet.
5 Bake in a preheated oven at 200°C (400°F) mark 6 for 15–20 minutes or until risen and golden brown. Dust with icing sugar and serve.

*H*OT CHOCOLATE MINT SOUFFLÉS

Serve these wickedly delicious chocolate mint soufflés after a virtuously low-calorie main course.

Serves 6

173 kcals per serving

150 ml (¼ pint) milk
12 After Eight mints
25 g (1 oz) butter or margarine

20 g (¾ oz) plain flour
25 g (1 oz) caster sugar
3 eggs, separated

1 Lightly grease six 150 ml ('/₄ pint) ramekin dishes. (There is no need to use a paper collar when preparing these mini soufflés; the mixture rises successfully without.) Put the milk in a small saucepan with the mints and heat gently, stirring, until evenly blended.

2 Melt the butter or margarine in a large heavy-based saucepan. Stir in the flour and cook for 1 minute, then remove from the heat and blend in the milk mixture. Bring to the boil, stirring all the time, and cook for 1 minute. Remove from the heat, cool slightly, then beat in the sugar and egg yolks.

3 Whisk the egg whites until stiff but not dry. Beat one spoonful into the sauce to lighten it, then gently fold in the remaining egg whites. Spoon into the prepared dishes.

4 Cook in a preheated oven at 190°C (375°F) mark 5 for 15–20 minutes or until set. Serve at once.

SUMMER PUDDING

Try to include some darker fruits such as blackcurrants, blackberries or raspberries to give the pudding a good colour.

Serves 6

130 kcals per serving

8 slices of day-old bread, crusts removed

225 g (8 oz) strawberries, hulled and halved if large

450 g (1 lb) mixed soft fruits, such as blackberries, redcurrants,

raspberries, loganberries and stoned cherries

75 ml (5 tbsp) apple juice

25 g (1 oz) sugar

Greek yogurt, to serve

1 Place one slice of bread in the base of a 900 ml (1¹/₂ pint) pudding basin. Reserve two slices of bread and use the remainder to line the sides of the basin, cutting them slightly to fit if necessary.

2 Put the fruit in a saucepan with the apple juice and sugar. Bring gently to the boil and cook for 2–3 minutes or until the fruit is slightly softened.

3 Fill the basin with the fruit, pressing it down well. Place the reserved bread on the top, cutting it to fit. Place a saucer on top of the pudding and weigh it down. Chill for at least 6 hours or overnight.

4 Just before serving, invert the pudding on to a large plate. Serve with Greek yogurt.

*P*EAR BAVARIAN CREAM

This is a deliciously smooth and refreshing dessert, with comparatively few calories.

Serves 8

132 kcals per serving

300 ml (½ pint) semi-skimmed milk
2 eggs, separated
50 g (2 oz) sugar
30 ml (2 tbsp) pear liqueur or brandy
15 ml (1 tbsp) powdered gelatine
1 ripe pear, peeled, cored and puréed
300 ml (10 fl oz) low-fat natura l
   yogurt

pear slices dipped in lemon juice, to
   decorate

For the Pear Sauce
1 ripe pear, peeled, cored and puréed
150 ml (¼ pint) unsweetened apple
   juice
10 ml (2 tsp) arrowroot

1   Lightly oil a 1.2 litre (2 pint) fluted mould and set aside. Warm the milk to just below boiling point. Put the egg yolks and sugar in a bowl and whisk until light and fluffy. Whisk in the milk until well blended. Return the mixture to the saucepan and heat gently, stirring, until thick enough to coat the back of a wooden spoon lightly. Set aside.

2   In a heatproof bowl, combine the liqueur or brandy with 30 ml (2 tbsp) water. Sprinkle the gelatine on to the liquid and leave to soak for 1 minute. Place over a pan of simmering water and stir until the gelatine is dissolved. Cool slightly.

3   Transfer the custard mixture to a bowl and stir in the pear purée and gelatine mixture. Place the bowl in a larger bowl filled with ice cubes and stir the mixture until it starts to thicken. Whisk the egg whites until stiff. Fold the yogurt and then the egg whites into the custard.

4   Pour the mixture into the prepared mould and chill for 2–3 hours or until set.

5   Meanwhile, place the sauce ingredients in a saucepan. Bring to the boil, stirring, and cook until slightly thickened and smooth. Leave to cool, stirring occasionally.

6   Turn out the mould and decorate with pear slices dipped in lemon juice. Serve with the pear sauce.

*M*INTED STRAWBERRY CUSTARDS

Replace the mint with a few lemon geranium leaves, if available, to produce a subtle and refreshing lemon flavour.

Serves 6

130 kcals per serving

450 ml (¾ pint) semi-skimmed milk
4 large sprigs of fresh mint
1 egg
2 egg yolks
45 ml (3 tbsp) caster sugar

20 ml (4 tsp) powdered gelatine
700 g (1½ lb) strawberries, hulled
artificial sweetener (optional)
strawberries, to decorate

1   Oil six 150 ml (¼ pint) ramekin dishes.
2   Place the milk and mint sprigs in a saucepan. Bring slowly to the boil, remove from the heat, cover and leave to infuse for about 30 minutes.
3   Whisk the egg and egg yolks with the caster sugar in a bowl. Strain over the milk. Return to the pan and cook gently, stirring, until the custard just coats the back of a wooden spoon. Do not boil. Leave to cool.
4   Sprinkle the gelatine over 45 ml (3 tbsp) water in a small heatproof bowl and leave to soak for 2–3 minutes. Place the bowl over a pan of simmering water and stir until dissolved. Stir the gelatine into the custard.
5   Purée and sieve the strawberries. Whisk about two thirds into the cold, but not set, custard. Pour the custard into the prepared dishes and chill for about 3 hours or until set.
6   Meanwhile, sweeten the remaining strawberry purée to taste with artificial sweetener, if desired. Chill.
7   To serve, turn out the custards. Surround with strawberry sauce, then decorate with strawberries.

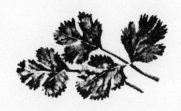

*C*OMPÔTE OF FRUIT WITH ELDERFLOWER CREAM

In this recipe, the fruit, which can include any varieties in season, is poached in fruit juice rather than a high-calorie sugar syrup. Elderflowers are beautifully aromatic and grow abundantly in the hedgerows. You can find dried elderflowers in health food shops.

Serves 4 or 6

250 or 167 kcals per serving

25 g (1 oz) sugar
6 large heads of fresh elderflowers or 25 g (1 oz) dried elderflowers
150 ml (5 fl oz) fresh double cream
900 g (2 lb) mixed fresh fruit, such as gooseberries, rhubarb, pears,

strawberries and cherries, prepared
300 ml (½ pint) unsweetened orange or apple juice
1 cinnamon stick
2 strips of lemon rind

1 To make the elderflower cream, put the sugar and 150 ml (¼ pint) water in a saucepan and heat gently until the sugar has dissolved, then boil rapidly until the liquid is reduced by half. Take off the heat and submerge the fresh or dried flowers in the syrup.
2 Leave to infuse for at least 2 hours, then press the syrup through a sieve, discarding the elderflowers. Whip the cream until it just holds its shape, then fold in the elderflower syrup. Chill until ready to serve.
3 Put the fruit, fruit juice, cinnamon and lemon rind in a large saucepan and simmer gently for 3–5 minutes or until the fruits are softened but still retain their shape. Remove the cinnamon and lemon rind and serve the compôte warm or cold with the elderflower cream.

*P*ASSION FRUIT SORBET WITH
MANGO SAUCE

Fructose is the type of sugar found in fruit. It is available in powdered or crystallized form from supermarkets.

Serves 4

160 kcals per serving

finely grated rind and juice of 2 limes
90 g (3½ oz) fructose (fruit sugar)
450 g (1 lb) passion fruit
2 egg whites

1 large ripe mango
30 ml (2 tbsp) orange juice
4 slices of lime, to decorate

1 Put the lime rind in a saucepan with 200 ml (7 fl oz) water and 75 g (3 oz) of the fructose. Stir over a low heat until the fructose has dissolved, then bring to the boil and simmer for 5 minutes. Leave to cool.

2 Halve the passion fruit and scoop out the seeds and flesh into a blender or food processor. Blend for a few seconds. Do not blend for too long or the seeds will be finely crushed and will add black specks to the sorbet. Rub the fruit through a fine sieve.

3 Strain the fructose syrup and combine with the strained passion fruit juice and lime juice. Stir well. Pour into a freezer tray or a 900 g (2 lb) loaf tin, cover and freeze until ice crystals begin to form around the edge.

4 Whisk the egg whites until foamy, add the remaining fructose and continue whisking until stiff.

5 Tip the partially frozen passion fruit mixture into a chilled bowl and whisk thoroughly. Fold in the egg whites and whisk lightly together. Return to the freezer tray or tin and freeze until firm.

6 To prepare the sauce, peel the mango and cut the flesh away from the stone. Put the flesh into a blender or food processor, add the orange juice and blend until smooth.

7 Serve the sorbet in glasses with the mango sauce spooned on top. Decorate each with a twist of lime.

BLACKCURRANT AND ROSE WATER MOUSSES

As an alternative, use redcurrants in this delicious light summer dessert.

Serves 4

100 kcals per serving

200 ml (7 fl oz) Greek yogurt
290 g (10½ oz) can blackcurrants in unsweetened fruit juice, drained and juice reserved

5 ml (1 tsp) rose water, plus a few drops
15 ml (1 tbsp) powdered gelatine
1 egg white

1 Put the yogurt in a bowl. Add 90 ml (6 tbsp) of the juice from the can of blackcurrants and 5 ml (1 tsp) rose water. Beat well together.

2 Sprinkle the gelatine over 60 ml (4 tbsp) cold water in a small heatproof bowl and leave to soak for 1 minute. Place over a pan of gently boiling water and stir until the gelatine is dissolved. Set aside to cool slightly, then stir into the yogurt mixture. Whisk the egg white until stiff and fold gently into the mixture.

3 Rinse the insides of four ramekin dishes with cold water and drain. Spoon in the yogurt mixture and level the surface. Chill for 2–3 hours or until set.

4 To serve, run a knife around the edge of each ramekin dish and turn out each mousse on to a plate. Carefully spoon the blackcurrants on top and sprinkle with a few drops of rose water. Serve immediately.

RASPBERRY BOMBE

This delicious and stunning-looking dessert requires only 25 ml (1½ tbsp) added sugar – use less if you wish.

Serves 4

75 kcals per serving

225 g (8 oz) raspberries, thawed if frozen
25 ml (1½ tbsp) sugar

10 ml (2 tsp) Crème de Cassis
225 g (8 oz) low-fat natural set yogurt
1 egg white, size 2

1 Put 175 g (6 oz) raspberries in a blender or food processor with half the sugar and the liqueur, and blend to make a purée. Reserve the remaining raspberries for decoration. Pour the purée into a freezerproof bowl and fold in the yogurt.
2 Put the bowl in the freezer for 1 hour or until ice crystals begin to form around the edge.
3 Whisk the egg white until stiff, then whisk in the remaining sugar and fold through the purée. Pour into a 900 ml (1½ pint) decorative freezerproof mould.
4 Return to the freezer and leave for at least 6 hours or until set. Stir at least once during this time.
5 To serve, turn the bombe out of the bowl and decorate with the reserved raspberries. Cut into slices.

*R*ED FRUIT GÂTEAU

A deliciously light dessert cake to capture the spirit of summer. Fromage frais makes an unusual low-calorie topping.

Serves 8 or 10

124 or 99 kcals per serving

For the Cake
3 eggs
75 g (3 oz) soft brown
  sugar
75 g (3 oz) plain flour
finely grated rind of 1 lemon

For the Filling and Decoration
450 g (1 lb) mixed summer fruit, such
  as raspberries, strawberries,
  redcurrants, loganberries and figs
100 g (4 oz) natural fromage frais
artificial sweetener

1 Grease and base-line two 18 cm (7 inch) sandwich tins. Grease the paper. Put the eggs and sugar in a large bowl. Using an electric whisk, beat the mixture until very thick and pale.
2 Carefully fold in the flour and lemon rind. Divide the mixture between the prepared tins. Bake in a preheated oven at 190°C (375°F) mark 5 for about 25 minutes. When cooked, the cake will look evenly brown, will spring back when lightly pressed, and will have shrunk slightly from the sides of the tins. Cool in the tins for 5 minutes, then turn out on to a wire rack and leave to cool completely.
3 To assemble the gâteau, sandwich the cakes together with most of the fruit, reserving some for decoration. Spread the fromage frais evenly over the top of the cake. Lightly sprinkle the remaining fruit with artificial sweetener and use to decorate the cake.

*F*LOATING SPICE ISLANDS

This dish consists of poached meringues floating on a blackcurrant sauce.

Serves 8

54 kcals per serving

For the Sauce
350 g (12 oz) blackcurrants, stalks
  removed
30 ml (2 tbsp) Crème de Cassis
artificial sweetener

For the Meringue
2 egg whites
50 g (2 oz) caster sugar
grated nutmeg
pinch of salt

1 To make the sauce, place the blackcurrants in a small saucepan with 60 ml (4 tbsp) water. Cover tightly and cook gently until the fruit softens. Rub through a nylon sieve, then leave to cool. Stir in the liqueur and sweeten to taste with artificial sweetener. Cover and chill.

2 Meanwhile, to make the meringue, whisk the egg whites in a bowl until stiff, but not dry. Gradually whisk in the caster sugar, keeping the mixture stiff. Fold in 1.25 ml ($^1/_4$ tsp) grated nutmeg.

3 Pour 2 cm ($^3/_4$ inch) water into a large frying pan and bring to a gentle simmer. Add the salt.

4 Shape the meringue into small egg shapes, using two spoons as a mould. Slide about six or eight at a time into the liquid and poach gently for 2–3 minutes. The meringue will puff up, then shrink back a little. When cooked, it will be firm if lightly touched. Remove with a fish slice and drain on absorbent kitchen paper. Poach the remaining mixture. Store in a cool place for not more than 2 hours.

5 To serve, spoon a little blackcurrant sauce on to individual serving dishes. Float a few 'islands' on top and sprinkle with nutmeg.

BETTER BAKING

*C*AKES, biscuits and buns don't have to be forbidden when you're on a diet. It's not a good idea to eat lots of them because, generally, they don't contain many nutrients. If you are on a calorie-reduced diet you can easily eat your way through thousands of calories worth of cakes and biscuits, without getting the protein, vitamins and minerals your body needs to keep going.

If eaten only occasionally, however, there's nothing wrong with a good slice of cake, a biscuit or a bun with a cup of coffee. In this chapter we show you how to achieve lower-calorie baking. For example, it's possible to reduce the sugar content by using naturally sweet fruits like sultanas, raisins, prunes and apples.

To increase your fibre intake, use half plain and half wholemeal flour, or even all wholemeal flour, when baking. Used in moderation, chopped nuts add flavour and texture to all baked goods, both sweet and savoury, and they are rich in protein and other nutrients. Spices and herbs add flavour and, in some recipes, can reduce the amount of salt or sugar needed.

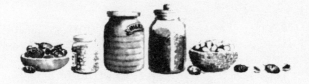

SESAME CRACKERS

Keep a batch of these easy-to-make biscuits on hand for a high-protein snack or lunch-box filler.

Makes 20

80 kcals per cracker

100 g (4 oz) plain wholemeal flour
100 g (4 oz) plain white flour
2.5 ml (½ tsp) baking powder
2.5 ml (½ tsp) bicarbonate of soda
45 ml (3 tbsp) sesame seeds

15 ml (1 tbsp) sugar
45 ml (3 tbsp) vegetable oil
50 g (2 oz) polyunsaturated margarine

1 Lightly grease a baking sheet and set aside. Sift together the flours, baking powder and bicarbonate of soda, adding any bran left in the sieve. Stir in the sesame seeds and sugar. Add the oil and margarine, then gradually add about 25 ml (1½ tbsp) water and mix to a smooth dough. Roll out on a lightly floured surface to about 0.5 cm (¼ inch) thick.
2 Cut out the biscuits with a 7.5 cm (3 inch) plain cutter. Place on the prepared baking sheet and bake in a preheated oven at 200°C (400°F) mark 6 for 15 minutes or until firm and slightly risen. Remove from the oven and leave to stand for 1 minute before transferring to a wire rack to cool. Store in an airtight container.

RYE CRISPBREADS

Rye flour is available from health food shops and most large supermarkets.

Makes 16

75 kcals per crispbread

225 g (8 oz) rye flour
5 ml (1 tsp) mustard powder
2.5 ml (½ tsp) caraway seeds
2.5 ml (½ tsp) paprika

salt and freshly ground pepper
50 g (2 oz) polyunsaturated
  margarine
105 ml (7 tbsp) semi-skimmed milk

1 Lightly grease two large baking sheets and set aside. Put the flour, mustard, caraway seeds, paprika and salt and pepper to taste in a bowl. Rub in the margarine until the mixture resembles fine breadcrumbs. Add the milk and mix to a firm dough.

2 Roll out the dough on a lightly floured surface to a 30 × 40 cm (12 × 16 inch) rectangle. Cut into 7.5 × 10 cm (3 × 4 inch) rectangles and place on the prepared baking sheets. Prick each rectangle several times with a fork to prevent rising during baking.

3 Bake in a preheated oven at 200°C (400°F) mark 6 for 10–15 minutes or until golden brown. Cool slightly on the baking sheets, then transfer to wire racks to cool. Store in an airtight container.

*G*INGERNUT BISCUITS

These spicy biscuits are always welcome as a teatime treat. These home-made gingernuts are lower in calories than the bought variety.

Makes 25

50 kcals per biscuit

90 g (3½ oz) plain wholemeal flour
90 g (3½ oz) self-raising wholemeal
  flour
15 ml (1 tbsp) ground ginger

65 g (2½ oz) butter or margarine
25 g (1 oz) sugar
65 ml (2½ fl oz) clear honey

1 Lightly grease two baking sheets and set aside. Put the flours together in a bowl, then add the ginger and mix well.

2 Put the butter or margarine, sugar and honey in a saucepan and heat gently, stirring, until the sugar has dissolved. Add the melted mixture to the flour and mix well. Leave to stand for 20 minutes.

3 Knead the dough on a lightly floured surface and roll out to 0.5 cm (¼ inch) thick. Stamp into rounds using a 5 cm (2 inch) cutter. Re-roll and cut the trimmings to make a total of 25–30 biscuits. Alternatively, divide up the mixture, roll into small balls and flatten well.

4 Place the biscuits on the prepared baking sheets and bake in a pre-heated oven at 180°C (350°F) mark 4 for 12–15 minutes or until pale golden brown.

5 Leave the biscuits to cool for a few minutes on the baking sheets, then transfer to a wire rack and leave until they are cold and have hardened.

*L*EMON AND GINGER SHORTBREAD

Use the finest side on your grater for the lemon rind, or the shortbread will be ruined by unpleasant lumps of rind.

Makes 16

95 kcals per piece

175 g (6 oz) plain wholemeal flour
100 g (4 oz) butter or margarine
5 ml (1 tsp) ground ginger

50 g (2 oz) sugar
very finely grated rind of 1 lemon

1 Put the flour in a bowl and rub in the butter or margarine until the mixture resembles fine breadcrumbs.
2 Stir in the ginger, sugar and lemon rind and knead to form a smooth dough. Turn on to a lightly floured surface and divide the dough in half.
3 Roll out each half to an 18 cm (7 inch) round and place on a baking sheet. Mark each round into eight portions and prick all over with a fork. Crimp the edges to decorate.
4 Bake in a preheated oven at 150°C (300°F) mark 2 for 35–45 minutes or until light golden brown. Leave to cool on the baking sheet, then cut into portions.

*P*RUNE AND CINNAMON BUNS

A sweet, sticky treat to eat on days when you are feeling like indulging yourself.

Makes 12

125 kcals per bun

225 g (8 oz) strong plain white flour
2.5 ml (½ tsp) easy-blend dried yeast
2.5 ml (½ tsp) salt
15 ml (1 tbsp) ground cinnamon
15 g (½ oz) butter or margarine
about 175 ml (6 fl oz) tepid semi-skimmed milk

175 g (6 oz) stoned prunes, roughly
  chopped
finely grated rind of 1 lemon
50 g (2 oz) soft light brown sugar
15 ml (1 tbsp) clear honey
15 ml (1 tbsp) lemon juice

1 Lightly grease and base-line an 18 cm (7 inch) square shallow cake tin.

2 Mix together the flour, dried yeast, salt and cinnamon. Rub in the butter or margarine, then beat in enough milk to mix to a soft dough.

3 Turn the dough on to a lightly floured surface and knead for about 5 minutes or until smooth. Place in a bowl, cover with a clean cloth and leave to rise in a warm place for about 1 hour or until doubled in size.

4 Knock back the dough and roll out to a 30 × 22.5 cm (12 × 9 inch) rectangle. Cover with the prunes and sprinkle over the lemon rind and sugar.

5 Roll up the dough from the longest edge like a Swiss roll and press down well to seal the edge. Cut into six thick slices and halve each slice diagonally. Place the slices, cut-side uppermost, in the prepared tin. Cover lightly with a clean cloth and leave to rise in a warm place for about 30 minutes or until the dough feels springy.

6 Bake the buns in a preheated oven at 190°C (375°F) mark 5 for about 30 minutes or until well risen and golden. Turn out of the tin on to a wire rack which is placed over a baking sheet. Gently remove the lining paper.

7 Mix the honey with the lemon juice and brush over the buns while still warm. Serve warm or cool or wrap loosely in aluminium foil and store in an airtight container for up to 2 days.

*B*LACKCURRANT MUFFINS

Of all fruit, blackcurrants are the richest source of vitamin C, some of which will still be present in these muffins after cooking.

Makes 12

90 kcals per muffin

100 g (4 oz) self-raising wholemeal flour
100 g (4 oz) self-raising white flour
75 g (3 oz) caster sugar
2 egg whites

75 g (3 oz) blackcurrants, thawed if frozen, stalks removed
200 ml (7 fl oz) semi-skimmed milk
60 ml (4 tbsp) vegetable oil

1 Lightly grease 12 muffin or patty tins and set aside. Mix together the flours and sugar. Lightly whisk the egg whites until they form soft peaks and add to the dry mixture with the remaining ingredients. Stir lightly.

2 Spoon the mixture into the tins and bake in a preheated oven at 200°C (400°F) mark 6 for 18–20 minutes or until the muffins are well risen and golden brown.

3 Serve immediately, or cool and reheat at 180°C (350°F) mark 4 for 5–6 minutes. Halve and serve spread with low-fat soft cheese.

SPICY APPLE AND COCONUT TARTS

Use firm, well-flavoured apples, such as Cox's, to make these delicious apple tarts.

Makes 12

130 kcals per tart

175 g (6 oz) plain flour
75 g (3 oz) butter or margarine
30 ml (2 tbsp) caster sugar
3 eating apples, cored and coarsely grated

50 g (2 oz) desiccated coconut
5 ml (1 tsp) ground mixed spice
2 egg whites

1 Lightly grease 12 patty tins and set aside. To make the pastry, put the flour in a bowl and rub in the butter or margarine until the mixture resembles fine breadcrumbs. Add 15 ml (1 tbsp) sugar and enough water (30–45 ml/2–3 tbsp) to form a smooth dough.
2 Turn the dough on to a lightly floured surface and roll out thinly. Using a 7.5 cm (3 inch) fluted cutter, cut out 12 rounds and use them to line the patty tins. Set aside.
3 Mix together the apples, coconut and mixed spice. Whisk the egg whites until lightly stiff, then fold gently into the apple mixture.
4 Divide the filling equally between the lined patty tins, packing the mixture down well. Sprinkle the remaining sugar evenly over the tarts.
5 Bake in a preheated oven at 190°C (375°F) mark 5 for 20–25 minutes or until the pastry is brown and the filling golden. Cool on a wire rack.

MIXED FRUIT TEABREAD

This very easy, foolproof recipe is ideal for family teas. It improves if kept for a day or two before cutting.

Makes 20 slices

90 kcals per slice

100 g (4 oz) raisins
100 g (4 oz) sultanas
50 g (2 oz) currants
100 g (4 oz) golden syrup
300 ml (½ pint) strained cold tea

1 egg, beaten
225 g (8 oz) plain wholemeal flour
7.5 ml (1½ tsp) baking powder
2.5 ml (½ tsp) ground mixed spice

1 Grease and base-line a 900 g (2 lb) loaf tin. Place the dried fruit and syrup in a large bowl. Pour over the tea, stir well to mix and leave to soak overnight.
2 The next day, add the egg, flour, baking powder and mixed spice to the fruit and tea mixture. Beat thoroughly with a wooden spoon until all the ingredients are evenly combined.
3 Spoon the mixture into the prepared tin and level the surface.
4 Bake in a preheated oven at 180°C (350°F) mark 4 for about 1¼ hours or until the teabread is well risen and a skewer inserted in the centre comes out clean.
5 Turn the teabread out of the tin and leave on a wire rack until completely cold. Wrap in cling film and store in an airtight container for 1–2 days before slicing and eating.

*C*OURGETTE TEABREAD

Try this unusual teabread for breakfast, toasted and spread with a little low-sugar jam.

Make 12 slices

135 kcals per slice

225 g (8 oz) plain wholemeal flour
75 g (3 oz) plain white flour
5 ml (1 tsp) baking powder
1.25 ml (¼ tsp) ground mace
1.25 ml (¼ tsp) ground mixed spice
finely grated rind of ½ orange
salt

150 ml (5 fl oz) low-fat natural yogurt
30 ml (2 tbsp) honey
2 eggs, beaten
225 g (8 oz) courgettes, trimmed and grated
50 g (2 oz) cashew nuts, chopped

1 Grease and base-line a 900 g (2 lb) loaf tin with greaseproof paper and set aside. Sift the flours, baking powder, mace and mixed spice into a large bowl, adding the bran left in the sieve. Stir in the orange rind and salt to taste.
2 Beat in the yogurt, honey and eggs, add the courgettes and chopped nuts, and mix well.
3 Transfer the mixture to the prepared tin. Bake in a preheated oven at 190°C (375°F) mark 5 for 1 hour. If the top of the bread starts to darken too much, cover with a piece of aluminium foil.
4 Turn the teabread out on to a wire rack. Cut into slices and serve while still warm, or cool completely, then store in an airtight container until ready to serve.

COTTAGE CHEESE AND BRAZIL NUT TEABREAD

This recipe uses cottage cheese instead of butter or margarine, reducing its calorie content quite considerably.

Makes 15 slices

150 kcals per slice

225 g (8 oz) natural cottage cheese
75 g (3 oz) sugar
225 g (8 oz) self-raising wholemeal flour
finely grated rind and juice of 1 lemon
2 eggs, beaten

75 ml (5 tbsp) semi-skimmed milk
75 g (3 oz) stoned dates, rinsed and roughly chopped
75 g (3 oz) Brazil nuts, chopped
6 whole Brazil nuts, to decorate
15 ml (1 tbsp) clear honey, to glaze

1 Grease and base-line a 900 g (2 lb) loaf tin and set aside. Put all the ingredients, except the whole Brazil nuts and honey, into a bowl and beat well together to make a mixture with a soft dropping consistency.
2 Spoon into the prepared tin and level the surface. Lightly press the whole Brazil nuts down the centre to decorate.
3 Bake in a preheated oven at 180°C (350°F) mark 4 for 50–60 minutes or until risen and golden brown, covering with greaseproof paper if the teabread is browning too quickly. Turn out and brush with the honey while still warm. Leave to cool on a wire rack. Serve cold.

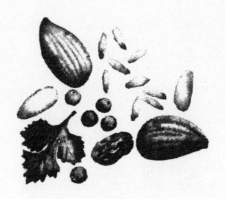

*H*AZELNUT CURRANT TWIST

This twisted loaf is rich in fibre, minerals and other nutrients, making it a healthy teatime treat.

Makes 12 slices

110 kcals per slice

150 ml (¼ pint) tepid semi-skimmed milk
50 g (2 oz) plus 5 ml (1 tsp) caster sugar
10 ml (2 tsp) dried yeast
175 g (6 oz) plain wholemeal flour
100 g (4 oz) strong plain white flour

2.5 ml (½ tsp) salt
5 ml (1 tsp) ground cinnamon
25 g (1 oz) butter or margarine, melted
25 g (1 oz) hazelnuts, chopped
50 g (2 oz) currants
honey, to glaze

1   Mix the milk with 5 ml (1 tsp) of the sugar and sprinkle the yeast over the mixture. Leave for 15 minutes, until frothy.

2   Mix together the wholemeal flour, plain flour, salt and cinnamon. Make a well in the centre and add the yeast liquid and melted butter or margarine. Mix to form a soft dough.

3   Turn the dough on to a lightly floured surface and knead for 5 minutes or until smooth and silky. Place in a bowl and cover with a clean cloth. Leave to rise for about 1 hour or until doubled in size.

4   Mix together the hazelnuts, the remaining sugar and the currants. Sprinkle the mixture, a little at a time, on to the dough, kneading it in until evenly mixed.

5   Divide the dough in half and shape into two 25 cm (10 inch) ropes. Twist the ropes together, pinching the ends to seal. Place on a baking sheet, cover with a clean cloth and leave to rise again for about 45 minutes or until the dough springs back when pressed.

6   Bake in a preheated oven at 190°C (375°F) mark 5 for 30–35 minutes or until the loaf is golden brown and sounds hollow when tapped on the base. Brush the top with a little honey while still warm, then leave to cool on a wire rack.

*H*AZELNUT AND CARROT CAKE

A light but very moist mixture, where the skins are left on the hazelnuts to add colour to the finished cake.

Makes 8 slices

99 kcals per slice

150 g (5 oz) hazelnuts with skins
3 eggs, separated
150 g (5 oz) caster sugar
225 g (8 oz) carrots, peeled and coarsely grated

finely grated rind of 1 lemon
50 g (2 oz) plain wholemeal flour
2.5 ml (½ tsp) baking powder
5 ml (1 tsp) ground mixed spice

1 Grease and base-line a 20 cm (8 inch) round, deep cake tin. Finely chop the hazelnuts, either by hand or in a food processor, taking care not to over-process or the nuts will become oily.

2 Place the egg yolks and sugar in a medium bowl and whisk until thick and pale. Stir in the nuts, carrots and lemon rind. Fold in the flour, baking powder and mixed spice.

3 Whisk the egg whites until stiff but not dry, and fold lightly into the cake mixture. Spoon into the prepared tin.

4 Bake in a preheated oven at 180°C (350°F) mark 4 for 40–50 minutes or until golden and springy to the touch.

5 Allow to cool in the tin for a few minutes before turning out on to a wire rack to cool completely. The cake can be stored in an airtight container for up to a week.

ENTERTAINING

IMPRESSIVE entertaining food doesn't have to consist of unhealthy, high-calorie dishes. Just because you are having a dinner party you don't have to stray from your calorie counting. There's no point in serving calorie-laden foods for your guests while you sit and suffer, because you're worrying about breaking your diet or because you can only eat a tiny portion. Serve a meal that you can eat and enjoy too.

In this chapter we give you nine well-balanced, calorie-counted meals. They are all less than 600 kcals for three courses, but that doesn't mean that they are unappetizing or boring. Your guests will never guess that they are eating so few calories – they'll all be delighted that they can enjoy such food without having to worry about their waistlines the next day!

Obviously, if you are trying to restrict yourself to just 1,000 calories per day, you will exceed the limit on an entertaining day. Don't worry, just try to redress the balance throughout the following week.

Keep accompaniments simple, such as a large mixed salad with the dressing handed separately (so you can add it sparingly, whilst your guests can be more generous), bread and butter where appropriate (limit yourself to just one slice without the butter) and lots of perfectly cooked vegetables.

Remember that alcohol will add lots of extra calories to your meal. If you can't go without, try to restrict your consumption by drinking spritzers or by alternating between wine and water. Always refill your own glass, so that you can keep a check on how much you are drinking.

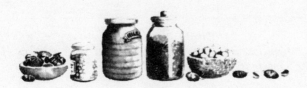

*D*INNER FOR EIGHT

514 kcals per person

Chicken Liver Pâté
Beef Olives with Mushroom Stuffing
Yogurt Brûlée

*C*HICKEN LIVER PÂTÉ

Serve this smooth pâté with plain Melba toast or warmed wholemeal pitta bread.

Serves 8

99 kcals per serving

25 g (1 oz) low-fat spread
1 medium onion, skinned and
    chopped
2 garlic cloves, skinned and crushed
450 g (1 lb) chicken livers, cleaned
    and dried

45 ml (3 tbsp) low-fat natural yogurt
15 ml (1 tbsp) tomato purée
15 ml (1 tbsp) brandy
salt and freshly ground pepper
pink peppercorns and fresh bay
    leaves, to garnish

1 Melt the low-fat spread in a heavy-based saucepan, add the onion and garlic and fry gently for 5 minutes. Add the chicken livers and cook for 5 minutes.
2 Remove from the heat and cool slightly, then add the yogurt, tomato purée, brandy and plenty of salt and pepper to taste.
3 Purée the mixture in a blender or food processor, then spoon into a serving dish. Chill for at least 2 hours, then serve garnished with peppercorns and bay leaves.

*Opposite: Prune and Cinnamon Buns (page 120);
Gingernut Biscuits (page 119); Blackcurrant Muffins (page (121)
Overleaf: Tea Cream with Cassis-Poached Fruits (page 139)*

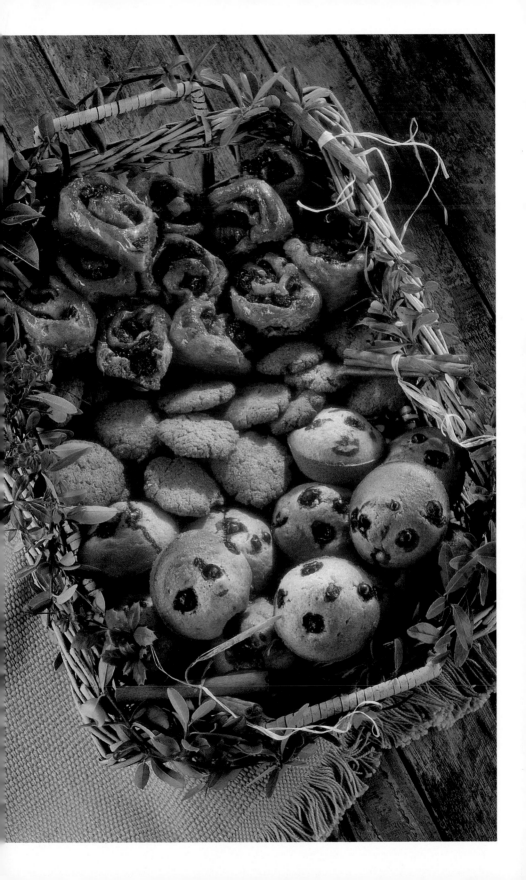

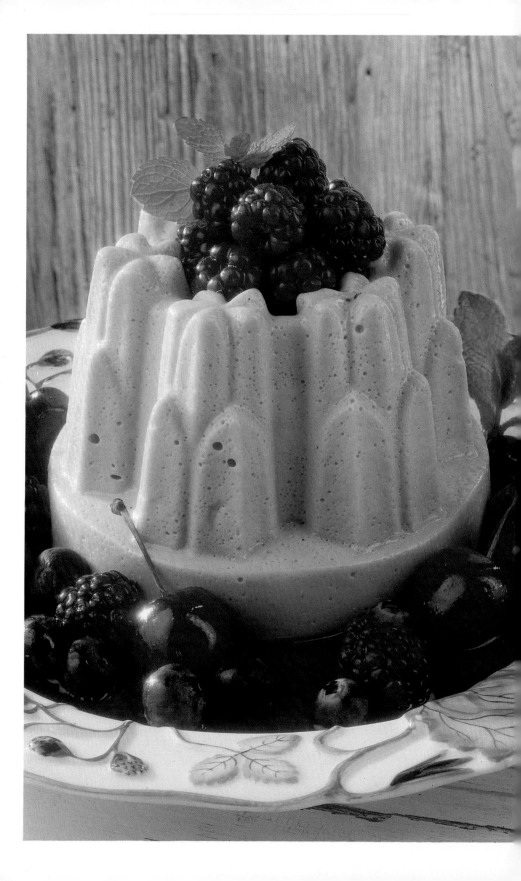

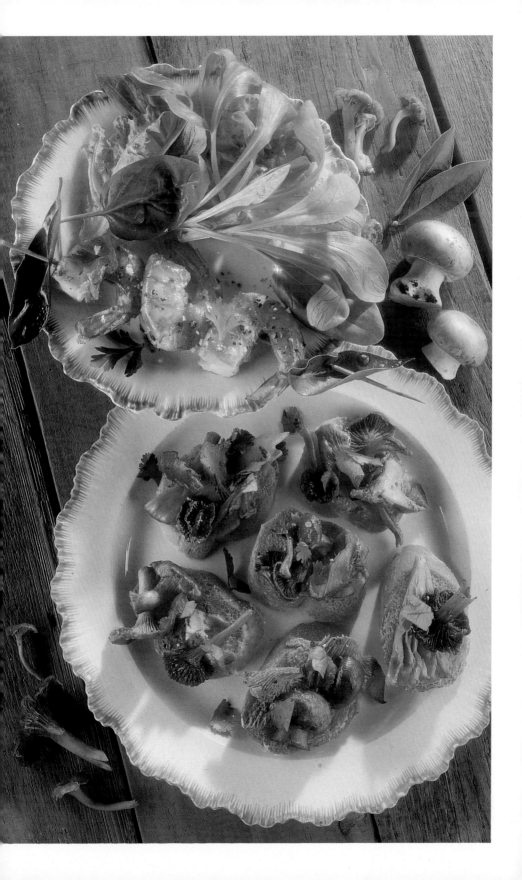

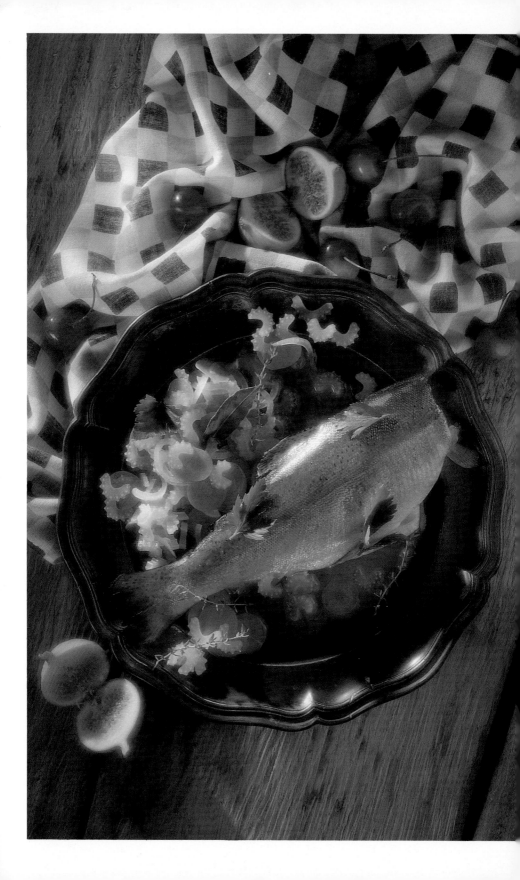

BEEF OLIVES WITH MUSHROOM STUFFING

Topside is one of the leaner cuts of beef, but be sure to trim off any visible fat before it is cooked. Serve with creamed garlic potatoes and a vegetable in season.

Serves 8

300 kcals per serving

16 thin slices of topside, each
weighing 75 g (3 oz)
25 g (1 oz) polyunsaturated margarine
300 ml (½ pint) dry red wine
salt and freshly ground pepper
30 ml (2 tbsp) tomato purée
finely chopped fresh parsley, to
garnish

For the Mushroom Stuffing
175 g (6 oz) button mushrooms, finely
chopped
10 ml (2 tsp) Dijon mustard
2 small carrots, scrubbed and grated
2 courgettes, trimmed and grated
30 ml (2 tbsp) breadcrumbs
15 ml (1 tbsp) tomato purée

1   Using a meat mallet or rolling pin, beat the beef slices between sheets of damp greaseproof paper until almost doubled in size.
2   To make the stuffing, mix together the mushrooms, mustard, carrot, courgette, breadcrumbs and tomato purée. Divide the mixture between the beef slices and spread evenly over. Roll up and secure at both ends with fine string.
3   Melt the margarine in a flameproof casserole and brown the prepared beef olives over a medium heat. Pour over the red wine and add salt and pepper to taste. Cover and cook for 45 minutes or until tender. Transfer the beef olives to a serving dish, discard the string and keep hot.
4   Skim the fat from the cooking liquid, then add the remaining tomato purée and adjust the seasoning. Heat through and pour over the beef olives. Garnish with parsley and serve at once.

Opposite: Trout Poached in Wine (page 147)
Previous page: Grilled Prawns with Garlic (page 134);
Baked Mushroom Croûtes (page 143)

YOGURT BRÛLÉE

Make this delicious fruit and yogurt brûlée in one large dish or in individual ramekins.

Serves 8

115 kcals per serving

225 g (8 oz) strawberries, hulled and halved

225 g (8 oz) raspberries, thawed if frozen

225 g (8 oz) redcurrants, thawed if frozen, stalks removed

30 ml (2 tbsp) Crème de Cassis

300 ml (½ pint) fat-reduced double cream substitute

300 ml (½ pint) Greek yogurt

25 g (1 oz) golden granulated sugar

1 Mix the prepared fruit with the liqueur in a flameproof serving dish. Set aside.

2 Whip the cream substitute until it forms soft peaks, then carefully fold in the yogurt. Spoon the mixture evenly over the fruit and smooth the surface. Cover and chill for at least 1 hour in the refrigerator.

3 To serve, sprinkle over the sugar and place under a preheated grill. Cook until brown and bubbling. Serve at once.

SUMMER LUNCH FOR EIGHT

461 kcals per person

Gazpacho
Dill-Glazed Salmon
Kiwi Fruit Sorbet

GAZPACHO

A traditional chilled Spanish soup, Gazpacho is quick to make and acts as an excellent appetite stimulant.

Serves 8

95 kcals per serving

450 g (1 lb) tomatoes, seeded and finely diced
½ a cucumber, peeled, seeded and finely diced
1 large onion, skinned and chopped
1 large green pepper, cored, seeded and diced
1 large red pepper, cored, seeded and diced
2 garlic cloves, skinned and finely chopped
900 ml (1½ pints) tomato juice, chilled

300 ml (½ pint) chicken or vegetable stock, chilled
30 ml (2 tbsp) olive oil
75 ml (5 tbsp) red wine vinegar
few drops of Tabasco sauce
salt and freshly ground pepper
45 ml (3 tbsp) chopped fresh chives or mint
2 slices of wholemeal bread, toasted and cubed, and ice cubes, to serve

1 Reserve about a quarter of the tomatoes, cucumber, onion and peppers for the garnish. Purée the remaining vegetables in a blender or food processor with the garlic and tomato juice until smooth.
2 Add the stock, oil, vinegar and Tabasco sauce and blend well. Season to taste with salt and pepper. Pour into a bowl, cover and chill for about 30 minutes.
3 Stir the soup and sprinkle with the fresh herbs. Serve with the reserved vegetables, wholemeal bread croûtons and ice cubes in separate bowls, to be added to the soup as desired.

DILL-GLAZED SALMON

For entertaining, a salmon looks impressive with its head and tail on. If this doesn't appeal or if you don't have a fish kettle or large enough roasting tin, the salmon will still make an excellent centrepiece with the head and tail removed. Serve with reduced-calorie mayonnaise, mixed half and half with low-fat natural yogurt and flavoured with chopped fresh dill. Steamed new potatoes and a herb and mixed leaf salad are the only other accompaniments needed.

Serves 8

291 kcals per serving

1.4 kg (3 lb) salmon or sea trout
dry white wine
onion and carrot slices, black
   peppercorns and bay leaf for
   flavouring

1 small bunch of fresh dill
2.5 ml (½ tsp) powdered gelatine
rocket or other green salad leaves
   and lemon and lime slices, to
   garnish

1 Rinse the salmon well under cold running water. Remove the head and tail, if wished. Place the salmon in a fish kettle or large roasting tin and pour over just enough cold water and a little dry white wine to cover. Add the flavouring ingredients and dill stalks. Divide the feathery dill tops into small sprigs, cover and refrigerate.

2 Cover the salmon with the kettle lid or foil. Bring the liquid slowly to the boil, then reduce the heat and simmer for 2 minutes. Turn off the heat and leave the salmon (still covered) in the liquid until cold.

3 Carefully remove the salmon from the poaching liquid. Strain and reserve 150 ml (¼ pint) of the liquid. Carefully skin the salmon, gently scraping away any dark brown flesh to reveal the pink underneath.

4 Place the salmon on a flat serving platter. If the head and tail are still on, cut a 'v' shape into the tail to neaten it. Cover the salmon with cling film and rerigerate for at least 30 minutes.

5 Place the reserved poaching liquid in a small bowl. Sprinkle over the powdered gelatine and leave to soak for 3–4 minutes. Place the bowl over a saucepan of simmering water and heat gently until the gelatine has completely dissolved. Cool the liquid until just beginning to thicken.

6 Brush a little of the thickened poaching liquid over the salmon. Press the reserved dill sprigs on to the exposed salmon flesh. Brush all over with more liquid. Return to the refrigerator to set.

7 To serve the salmon, garnish with a little rocket or other green salad leaves, and lemon and lime slices.

*K*IWI FRUIT SORBET

Strawberries make a delicious and colourful accompaniment to this refreshing dessert.

Serves 8

75 kcals per serving

100 g (4 oz) sugar
14 kiwi fruit

3 egg whites

1 Chill a shallow freezer container. Place the sugar in a heavy-based saucepan and pour over 150 ml ('/₄ pint) water. Warm over a low heat until the sugar has dissolved, then simmer for 2 minutes to form a syrup. Remove from the heat and leave to cool for 30 minutes.
2 Thinly peel 12 of the kiwi fruit and halve. Purée in a blender or food processor with the syrup, then pass through a nylon sieve to remove the pips. Freeze for 2 hours or until half-frozen.
3 Whisk the egg whites until just stiff, then fold into the half-frozen syrup until it is an even texture. Cover the freezer container and freeze for 4 hours or until firm. Remove from the freezer just before serving and spoon into glasses. Peel and slice the remaining kiwi fruit and use to decorate the sorbets.

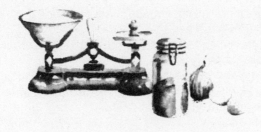

*E*XOTIC DINNER FOR SIX

488 kcals per person

Grilled Prawns with Garlic
Spiced Chicken with Cashew Nuts
Exotic Fruit Salad

*G*RILLED PRAWNS WITH GARLIC

For this recipe it is absolutely essential to buy giant prawns, which are only usually available at good fishmongers.

Serves 6

134 kcals per serving

24 frozen raw Pacific prawns or
   frozen Dublin Bay prawn tails,
   thawed
18 fresh bay leaves
75 g (3 oz) low-fat spread
3 large garlic cloves, skinned and
   crushed

15 ml (1 tbsp) chopped fresh oregano
   or 5 ml (1 tsp) dried
45 ml (3 tbsp) lemon juice
salt and freshly ground pepper
60 ml (4 tbsp) chopped fresh parsley,
   to garnish
lemon or lime wedges, to serve

1 If using Pacific prawns, remove the legs and with a sharp knife, make a slit down the centre of the back and remove the intestinal vein. Wash well. If using Dublin Bay prawn tails, make a slit through the shell on either side of the underside. Wash well.
2 Thread the prawns and bay leaves on to six skewers and place in a single layer on a well-oiled grill-pan.
3 Melt the low-fat spread in a saucepan, add the garlic and fry gently until golden. Remove from the heat and stir in the oregano, lemon juice and salt and pepper to taste.
4 Pour the garlic mixture over the prawns, turning them to coat well. Cook under a preheated grill for 5–8 minutes or until the prawns turn pink. Arrange on a warmed serving platter, pour over the pan juices and sprinkle with chopped parsley. Serve hot, with lemon or lime wedges.

SPICED CHICKEN WITH CASHEW NUTS

Serve with plain boiled rice and steamed fresh vegetables, such as broccoli or courgettes.

Serves 6

244 kcals per serving

6 chicken breast fillets, skinned
15 g (½ oz) fresh root ginger, peeled and roughly chopped
5 ml (1 tsp) coriander seeds
4 cloves
10 ml (2 tsp) black peppercorns
300 ml (10 fl oz) low-fat natural yogurt
1 medium onion, skinned and roughly chopped

50 g (2 oz) cashew nuts
2.5 ml (½ tsp) chilli powder
10 ml (2 tsp) ground turmeric
15 ml (1 tbsp) vegetable oil
salt
cashew nuts, chopped and toasted, and chopped fresh coriander, to garnish

1   Make shallow slashes with a sharp knife across each of the chicken breasts.
2   Put the ginger in a blender or food processor with the coriander seeds, cloves, peppercorns and yogurt and blend to a paste.
3   Pour the yogurt mixture over the chicken, cover and leave to marinate for about 24 hours, turning the chicken once.
4   Put the onion in a blender or food processor with the cashew nuts, chilli powder, turmeric and 150 ml (¼ pint) water. Blend to a paste.
5   Lift the chicken out of the marinade. Heat the oil in a large sauté pan, add the chicken pieces and fry until browned on both sides.
6   Stir in the marinade with the nut mixture and bring slowly to the boil. Season to taste with salt. Cover the pan and simmer for about 20 minutes or until the chicken is tender, stirring occasionally. Taste and adjust the seasoning and garnish with cashews and coriander before serving.

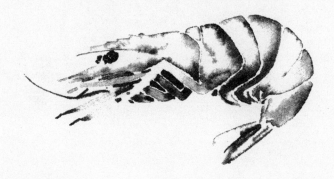

*E*XOTIC FRUIT SALAD

All these tropical fruits should be available at large supermarkets. You can add or substitute others.

Serves 6

110 kcals per serving

900 g (2 lb) ripe pineapple	1 passion fruit or pomegranate
1 mango or small papaya	4 lychees or rambutans
1 guava or banana, peeled and sliced	1 kiwi fruit

1　Cut the pineapple in half lengthways, with the leaves attached. Remove the core in a wedge from each half and discard. Cut out the flesh, cut into small chunks and place in a bowl. Scrape out the remaining flesh and juice with a spoon and add to the bowl. Reserve the empty halves of skin.

2　Peel the mango or papaya and discard the stone or seeds. Cut the flesh into cubes and add to the pineapple with the guava or banana.

3　Cut the passion fruit or pomegranate in half, and scoop out the seeds with a teaspoon. Add the seeds to the pineapple.

4　Peel the lychees or rambutans and cut in half. Remove the stones and add to the bowl of fruit.

5　Peel the kiwi fruit and cut the flesh into round slices. Add to the bowl of fruit and stir.

6　Spoon the fruit salad into the pineapple halves. Cover and chill until required.

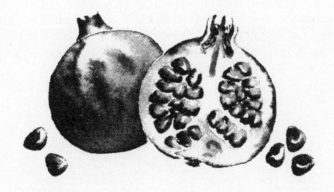

*I*NFORMAL SUPPER FOR SIX

598 kcals per person

Carrot and Garlic Dip
Smoked Mussel Steaks
Tea Cream with Cassis-Poached Fruits

*C*ARROT AND GARLIC DIP

Everyone loves to scoop up mouthfuls of a smooth dip on pieces of crunchy raw vegetable. Here, a purée of cooked carrot is blended with creamy natural yogurt and lightly spiced to make a very more-ish mixture.

Serves 6

65 kcals per serving

350 g (12 oz) carrots, scrubbed and sliced
1–2 garlic cloves, skinned and crushed
300 ml (10 fl oz) low-fat natural yogurt
2.5 ml (½ tsp) ground coriander

salt
selection of raw fresh vegetables, such as celery, red and green peppers, courgettes, radishes and cauliflower, cut into neat pieces or strips

cayenne

1   Cook the carrots in boiling salted water until just tender. Drain thoroughly, refresh with cold water and drain again.
2   Put the carrots in a blender or food processor with the garlic, yogurt and coriander and purée until smooth. Season generously with cayenne and a little salt. Turn into a serving dish and leave for about 1 hour to let the flavours develop. Serve with the vegetables.

SMOKED MUSSEL STEAKS

Serve with halved tomatoes, grilled and topped with parsley, and a large mixed salad.

Serves 6

325 kcals per serving

6 sirloin steaks, each weighing about 175 g (6 oz), and 2 cm (¾ inch) thick
105 g (3⅔ oz) can smoked mussels

30 ml (2 tbsp) white wine vinegar
1 bunch of watercress
salt and freshly ground pepper

1   Trim the steaks of any excess fat. With a sharp knife, make a horizontal slit along the length of each steak to form a pocket.

2   Drain the mussels, reserving the oil. Chop the mussels roughly and place in a bowl with the wine vinegar.

3   Trim the root ends off the watercress and chop roughly. Stir into the mussels with plenty of salt and pepper.

4   Spoon a little of the mussel mixture into each steak. Place in a single layer in a shallow flameproof dish, or on a foil-lined grill pan. Preheat the grill to hot.

5   Brush the steaks with the reserved oil from the mussels. Cook under the preheated grill for about 3–4 minutes on each side for a medium steak, about 5–6 minutes for well done. Turn the steaks over carefully with tongs or a fish slice to prevent the filling dropping out. Serve hot.

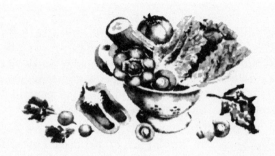

*T*EA CREAM WITH CASSIS-POACHED FRUITS

This delicately flavoured tea cream mould is perfectly complemented by the strong flavour and rich colour of the red fruit mixture.

Serves 6

208 kcals per serving

300 ml (½ pint) semi-skimmed milk
4 Earl Grey tea bags
2 eggs
15 ml (1 tbsp) sugar
15 g (½ oz) powdered gelatine
150 ml (5 fl oz) whipping cream, lightly whipped
150 ml (5 fl oz) low-fat natural yogurt

450 g (1 lb) mixed red fruits, such as cherries, redcurrants, boysenberries, blueberries and raspberries
300 ml (½ pint) unsweetened apple juice
artificial sweetener
30 ml (2 tbsp) Crème de Cassis
fresh mint, to decorate

1   Heat the milk to just below boiling point. Pour over the tea bags, cover and leave to infuse for 15–20 minutes. Squeeze the tea bags and discard.

2   Separate 1 egg, reserving the white. Beat the yolk with the remaining whole egg and the sugar. Add to the milk, beating well. Strain into a double saucepan or heavy-based pan. Cook over a gentle heat, stirring, until the custard thickens and coats the back of a wooden spoon, taking care not to let the custard curdle. Remove from the heat and cool.

3   Sprinkle the gelatine over 45 ml (3 tbsp) cold water in a heatproof bowl and leave to soak for 1 minute. Place over a pan of gently boiling water and stir until the gelatine is dissolved. Leave to cool slightly, then stir into the custard.

4   When just beginning to set, stir in the cream, then the yogurt. Whisk the reserved egg white until stiff and fold into the mixture. Pour into a dampened 900 ml (1½ pint) mould and chill for 2–3 hours or until set.

5   Meanwhile, make the fruit sauce. Prepare the fruit, removing any stones, as necessary. Put the fruit and apple juice with sweetener to taste in a saucepan and simmer gently until softened but still retaining some shape. Cool, then stir in the Cassis.

6   Unmould the tea cream by dipping quickly into very hot water and inverting on to a serving dish. Surround the tea cream with the poached fruits and serve at once, decorated with mint.

SUMMER LUNCH FOR SIX

424 kcals per person

Mushrooms Marinated with Crushed Coriander
Lamb Cutlets with Asparagus Sauce
Apple Mint Meringues

*M*USHROOMS MARINATED WITH CRUSHED CORIANDER

Serve these mushrooms with good bread to mop up the juices. Two slices of French bread will add about 100 kcals to the meal.

Serves 6

32 kcals per serving

30 ml (2 tbsp) coriander seeds
1–2 garlic cloves, skinned and
crushed
150 ml (¼ pint) dry red wine

700 g (1½ lb) small button
mushrooms, wiped
salt and freshly ground pepper
chopped fresh coriander, to garnish

1 Crush the coriander seeds using a pestle and mortar. Put them in a large saucepan with the garlic and wine and bring to the boil. Simmer for 5 minutes.
2 Add the mushrooms and cook gently for 3–4 minutes or until the mushrooms are tender. Remove from the heat and leave to cool. Season to taste with salt and pepper.
3 Leave to marinate overnight. Serve cold, garnished with coriander.

*L*AMB CUTLETS WITH ASPARAGUS SAUCE

If you grow your own asparagus, or have a friend who does, this is a good way of using up any awkwardly-sized spears.

Serves 6

263 kcals per serving

18 fresh asparagus spears, scraped and with ends trimmed
40 g (1½ oz) low-fat spread
1 onion, skinned and chopped

450 ml (¾ pint) chicken or vegetable stock
salt and freshly ground pepper
12 lamb cutlets, trimmed of all fat

1   Cut off the asparagus tips and reserve, then slice the stalks. Melt the low-fat spread in a saucepan, add the onion and asparagus stalks and cook gently for 5 minutes. Add the stock and salt and pepper to taste, bring to the boil, lower the heat, cover and simmer for 20 minutes or until tender. Leave to cool slightly, then purée the mixture in a blender or food processor until smooth. Return to the pan to reheat, and adjust the seasoning.
2   Grill the lamb cutlets for 10–15 minutes, turning once, until cooked as desired. Meanwhile, cook the reserved asparagus tips in boiling water for 5 minutes or until just tender. Drain and keep warm.
3   Serve the chops with the asparagus tips on a bed of asparagus sauce. Serve the remaining sauce separately.

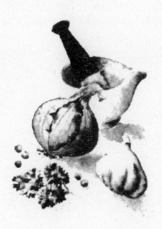

*A*PPLE MINT MERINGUES

The meringue rounds can be made well in advance and stored in an airtight container.

Serves 6

129 kcals per serving

2 egg whites
100 g (4 oz) caster sugar
350 g (12 oz) tart eating apples
15 ml (1 tbsp) artificial sweetener
4 sprigs of fresh mint

150 ml (5 fl oz) Greek yogurt
15 ml (1 tbsp) icing sugar, sprigs of
fresh mint and apple slices, to
decorate

1 Whisk the egg whites until stiff but not dry. Add 30 ml (2 tbsp) caster sugar and whisk again until stiff and shiny. Fold in the remaining sugar.

2 Mark twelve 7.5 cm (3 inch) rounds on a sheet of non-stick baking parchment. Divide the meringue mixture among the rounds and spread with a round-bladed knife to fill. Alternatively, using a 0.5 cm ($^{1}/_{4}$ inch) plain nozzle, pipe the mixture into the rounds. Bake in a preheated oven at 140°C (275°F) mark 1 for about 1 hour or until completely dried out and crisp. Leave to cool on a wire rack.

3 Peel, core and thinly slice the apples. Place in a saucepan with the artificial sweetener, four sprigs of mint and 30 ml (2 tbsp) water. Cover and cook very gently for about 10 minutes or until the apple has softened. Leave to cool, then cover and chill for at least 1 hour.

4 To serve, spoon a little apple on to six meringue rounds. Top with the yogurt and the remaining meringues. Dust lightly with icing sugar and decorate with sprigs of fresh mint and apple slices before serving.

SUPPER FOR SIX

499 kcals per person

Baked Mushroom Croûtes
Pissaladière
Lemon Muesli Cheesecake

BAKED MUSHROOM CROÛTES

Wild mushrooms give the best flavour, but if they are unavailable use all button mushrooms or the large flat mushrooms.

Serves 6

113 kcals per serving

225 g (8 oz) button mushrooms
225 g (8 oz) wild mushrooms, such as chanterelles, ceps, etc
30 ml (2 tbsp) roughly chopped fresh coriander
30 ml (2 tbsp) lemon juice
30 ml (2 tbsp) olive oil

salt and freshly ground pepper
6 thin slices of French bread
1 garlic clove, skinned and halved
25 g (1 oz) low-fat spread
roughly chopped fresh coriander, to garnish

1 Thinly slice the button mushrooms and any large wild ones. Place in an ovenproof dish and sprinkle over half the coriander, the lemon juice and the olive oil. Season to taste with salt and pepper.

2 Cover the dish with foil and bake in a preheated oven at 200°C (400°F) mark 6 for about 40 minutes. Stir the mixture once, halfway through the cooking time.

3 Rub the bread slices with the halved garlic clove. Thinly spread one side of each slice with low-fat spread. Arrange the slices, fat-side uppermost, in an ovenproof dish and bake in the oven for 10 minutes.

4 Spoon the hot mushrooms and juices over the six bread slices. Return to the oven for 15 minutes, then serve garnished with coriander and lemon wedges.

*P*ISSALADIÈRE

To keep the calorie content of this flan low, use just a few anchovies, well drained and sliced lengthways, and olives in brine to garnish.

Serves 6

170 kcals per serving

100 g (4 oz) plain flour
salt and freshly ground pepper
50 g (2 oz) butter or margarine
15 ml (1 tbsp) olive oil
450 g (1 lb) onions, skinned and finely
  sliced
2 garlic cloves, skinned and crushed

225 g (8 oz) tomatoes, skinned
30 ml (2 tbsp) tomato purée
5 ml (1 tsp) chopped fresh herbs,
  such as marjoram, thyme or sage
anchovy fillets, stoned black olives
  and parsley, to garnish

1 To make the pastry, put the flour in a bowl with a pinch of salt. Cut the butter or margarine into pieces and add to the flour.
2 Rub the fat into the flour until the mixture resembles fine bread-crumbs. Gradually add about 30 ml (2 tbsp) water, adding only enough to bind the mixture to a smooth dough. Wrap and chill in the refrigerator for 15 minutes.
3 When the dough is cool, turn on to a lightly floured surface and roll out very thinly. Use to line a 20.5 cm (8 inch) plain flan ring. Bake blind in a preheated oven at 200°C (400°F) mark 6 for 20 minutes.
4 Meanwhile, make the filling. Heat the oil in a heavy-based saucepan. Add the onions and garlic and fry for 2–3 minutes. Cover the pan with a tightly fitting lid, reduce the heat and cook for about 10 minutes or until the onions are very soft, but not brown. Shake the pan occasionally during cooking.
5 Slice the tomatoes, add to the pan and continue cooking, uncovered, for 10 minutes or until the liquid has evaporated. Stir in the tomato purée, herbs and salt and pepper to taste.
6 Turn the mixture into the flan case. Brush with a little oil and cook in the oven at 200°C (400°F) mark 6 for 20 minutes.
7 To serve, garnish the pissaladière with anchovy fillets, olives and parsley. Serve either hot or cold.

*L*EMON MUESLI CHEESECAKE

Make sure that you use a sugar-free muesli or the calories in this cheese-cake will be very high. Use half a chocolate flake to decorate the top if you prefer.

Serves 6

216 kcals per serving

175 g (6 oz) sugar-free muesli
75 g (3 oz) low-fat spread, melted
finely grated rind and juice of 2
    lemons
1 sachet (scant 15 ml/1 tbsp)
    powdered gelatine

225 g (8 oz) low-fat soft cheese
150 ml (¼ pint) low-fat natural yogurt
60 ml (4 tbsp) clear honey
2 egg whites
25 g (1 oz) plain chocolate

1 Mix the muesli and melted fat together. With the back of a metal spoon, press the mixture over the base of a greased 20.5 cm (8 inch) springform cake tin. Chill in the refrigerator to set while making the filling.
2 Make up the lemon juice to 150 ml (¼ pint) with water. Pour into a heatproof bowl.
3 Sprinkle the gelatine over the lemon juice and leave to stand for 5 minutes until spongy. Stand the bowl in a pan of hot water and heat gently, stirring occasionally, until the gelatine is dissolved. Set aside to cool slightly.
4 Whisk the cheese, yogurt and honey together in a separate bowl. Stir in the grated lemon rind and cooled gelatine.
5 Whisk the egg whites until standing in stiff peaks. Fold into the filling mixture until evenly incorporated. Spoon on top of the muesli base and level the surface. Chill in the refrigerator for at least 4 hours or until set.
6 To make the decoration, break the chocolate into small pieces and melt in a heatproof bowl set over a pan of gently simmering water. Spoon into a piping bag made from a sheet of greaseproof paper and drizzle over the top of the cheesecake. Leave to set.

DINNER FOR EIGHT

402 kcals per person

Parma Ham with Fruit
Trout Poached in Wine
Iced Rose Petal Soufflés

PARMA HAM WITH FRUIT

A simple, yet stunning start to a meal, this is a variation of a traditional Italian combination of melon and Parma ham.

Serves 8

50 kcals per serving

a selection of fresh fruits, including exotic fruits such as lychees, rambutans and figs

16 very thin slices of Parma ham (prosciutto)

Prepare the fruits as necessary and arrange attractively with the ham on eight serving plates.

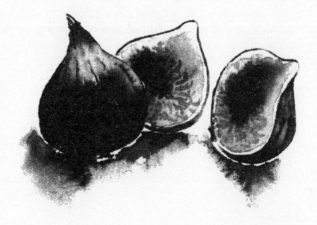

*T*ROUT POACHED IN WINE

This flavoursome trout dish is cooked with vegetables and therefore needs little accompaniment other than boiled new potatoes or crusty French bread.

Serves 8

210 kcals per serving

8 whole small trout, cleaned
salt and freshly ground pepper
25 g (1 oz) low-fat spread
1 large onion, skinned and sliced
4 celery sticks, trimmed and sliced
4 carrots, peeled and very thinly
    sliced

300 ml (½ pint) dry white wine
300 ml (½ pint) fish stock
bouquet garni
lemon wedges and chopped fresh
    parsley, to garnish

1   Wash the trout under cold running water and drain. Pat dry and season the insides.
2   Melt the low-fat spread in a small saucepan. Add the onion, celery and carrots and stir well to coat with fat. Cover and sweat for 5 minutes.
3   Lay the vegetables in a large casserole and arrange the fish on top. Pour over the wine and stock and add the bouquet garni.
4   Cover tightly and cook in a preheated oven at 180°C (350°F) mark 4 for about 25 minutes or until the trout are cooked.
5   Transfer to a warmed serving dish and keep hot.
6   Pour the cooking juices into a small pan, discarding the bouquet garni, and boil rapidly until reduced by half. Pour into a sauceboat or jug. Garnish with lemon and parsley.

*I*CED ROSE PETAL SOUFFLÉS

You can either make individual soufflés or one large one. Do not make more than two or three days in advance.

Serves 8

142 kcals per serving

50 g (2 oz) well scented rose petals, dried
100 g (4 oz) caster sugar
200 g (7 oz) low-fat soft cheese

75 g (3 oz) crème fraîche
few drops of rose water (optional)
4 egg whites
small rose petals, to decorate

1 Tie a double strip of greaseproof paper around eight 150 ml ($^1/_4$ pint) ramekin dishes to make 7.5 cm (3 inch) collars. Lightly brush the inside of the paper with oil.

2 Blend the rose petals and sugar in a blender or food processor until the petals are reduced to very small pieces.

3 Mix the low-fat soft cheese and crème fraîche together. Taste and add a few drops of rose water to increase the flavour, if necessary.

4 Whisk the egg whites until stiff but not dry, then gently fold into the cheese mixture with the sugared rose petals.

5 Divide the mixture between the prepared dishes. Freeze until firm, then cover the tops.

6 About 25 minutes before serving, remove the soufflés from the freezer and carefully ease away the paper collars. Leave the soufflés in the refrigerator until required. Serve decorated with small rose petals.

SUMMER DINNER FOR FOUR

591 kcals per person

Salad of Baked Goats' Cheese and Hazelnuts
Apricot and Redcurrant-Stuffed Pork
Honeydew Granita

SALAD OF BAKED GOATS' CHEESE AND HAZELNUTS

Include some of the newly-available lettuce leaves, such as oakleaf, frisée or radicchio to make this a very attractive starter.

Serves 4

241 kcals per serving

25 g (1 oz) hazelnuts
12 thin slices of French bread
12 thin slices of goats' cheese
mixed salad leaves

10 ml (2 tsp) hazelnut oil
45 ml (3 tbsp) low-calorie vinaigrette
freshly ground pepper

1 Place the hazelnuts on a baking sheet and toast in a preheated oven at 180°C (350°F) mark 4 for 10–12 minutes or until thoroughly browned. Tip the nuts on to a clean tea-towel and rub off the loose skins. Roughly chop the nuts, then return to the oven for 2–3 minutes or until evenly browned.
2 Increase the oven temperature to 220°C (425°F) mark 7. Arrange the slices of French bread on a baking sheet. Top each with a slice of cheese and bake for 10 minutes or until the bread is crisp and the cheese hot but not melted.
3 Meanwhile, arrange the salad leaves on six plates. Whisk the hazelnut oil into the low-calorie vinaigrette.
4 When the cheese and bread are ready, arrange on top of the salad leaves. Sprinkle each with a little of the dressing and the hazelnuts. Grind a little pepper over the top and serve immediately.

APRICOT AND REDCURRANT- STUFFED PORK

Serve this deliciously fruity pork dish garnished with extra redcurrants and plenty of parsley.

Serves 4

265 kcals per serving

25 g (1 oz) brown rice
one 550–700 g (1¼–1½ lb) pork fillet (tenderloin), trimmed of all fat
½ small onion, skinned and chopped
50 g (2 oz) redcurrants, thawed if frozen, stalks removed
100 g (4 oz) apricots, stoned and chopped

1 small cooking apple, peeled, cored and chopped
finely grated rind of 1 small orange
30 ml (2 tbsp) chopped fresh parsley
salt and freshly ground pepper
30 ml (2 tbsp) orange juice
5 ml (1 tsp) sugar-free apricot jam

1 Add the rice to 150 ml (¼ pint) boiling water. Reduce the heat, cover and simmer for 30 minutes or until the rice is just tender and the liquid is absorbed.

2 Meanwhile, split open the pork fillet lengthways, without cutting it in half. Spread the meat out flat, cut-side down, cover with greaseproof paper and pound with a flat mallet to form a 30×20 cm (12×8 inch) rectangle.

3 Put the onion in a bowl with the redcurrants, apricots, apple, orange rind, 15 ml (1 tbsp) chopped parsley, cooked rice and salt and pepper to taste. Mix well.

4 Spoon the stuffing over the pork fillet and spread to within 4 cm (1½ inches) of the edge. Fold over the two short ends of the pork fillet, then roll up, Swiss-roll fashion, from a long side. Tie the roll with string at 4 cm (1½ inch) intervals.

5 Place the meat on a piece of aluminium foil and spoon over 15 ml (1 tbsp) orange juice. Wrap the foil loosely around the meat and seal across the top. Place on a baking sheet. Cook at 190°C (375°F) mark 5 for 45 minutes. Fold back the foil, baste the meat with the cooking juices and cook for a further 10 minutes.

6 Remove the meat from the foil and keep warm on a serving plate. Pour the juices from the foil into a saucepan and add the remaining orange juice and the jam. Bring to the boil and cook until reduced by half. Strain, then stir in the remaining parsley.

7 Remove the string and serve the meat, cut into slices, with a little sauce poured over. Serve the remaining sauce separately.

*H*ONEYDEW GRANITA

A light honey, such as Acacia, is recommended for this dish as a strong-flavoured honey may mask the flavour of the melon.

Serves 4

85 kcals per serving

1.4–1.6 kg (3–3½ lb) honeydew melon, peeled, seeded and cut into chunks
15 ml (1 tbsp) clear honey

finely grated rind and juice of 1 small orange
finely grated rind and juice of 1 lemon
sprigs of fresh mint, to garnish

1 Purée the melon in a blender or food processor, then place in a bowl with the honey, orange and lemon rind and juice. Mix well.
2 Transfer the mixture to a rigid freezerproof container and freeze for 3 hours or until the mixture is partly frozen and setting around the edges.
3 Turn the mixture into a bowl and whisk well to break up the ice crystals. Freeze for about 4 hours or until frozen. Before serving, soften the granita in the refrigerator for about 45 minutes. Spoon into chilled glasses or dishes and garnish with mint sprigs.

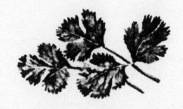

*D*INNER FOR SIX

562 kcals per person

Tomato Ice with Vegetable Julienne
Monkfish Thermidor
Figs with Raspberry Sauce

*T*OMATO ICE WITH VEGETABLE JULIENNE

Serve this unusual first course with Melba toast to make a refreshingly light starter, ideal for serving before the richly flavoured monkfish dish.

Serves 6

137 kcals per serving

8 very ripe tomatoes
10 ml (2 tsp) powdered gelatine
30 ml (2 tbsp) tomato purée
30 ml (2 tbsp) lemon juice or juice of
  ½ lemon
few drops of Tabasco sauce
salt and freshly ground pepper
30 ml (2 tbsp) chopped fresh basil

1 egg white (optional)
2 small leeks, trimmed
2 medium carrots, scrubbed
2 medium courgettes, trimmed
150 ml (¼ pint) low-calorie vinaigrette
fresh basil leaves, to garnish

1   Put the tomatoes in a blender or food processor and blend until smooth. Press the tomato pulp through a sieve into a bowl.
2   Put 45 ml (3 tbsp) very hot water in a small bowl and sprinkle in the gelatine. Stir briskly until dissolved, then leave to cool slightly.
3   Add the tomato purée to the tomato pulp with the lemon juice, Tabasco and salt and pepper to taste. Mix thoroughly.
4   Stir in the gelatine and chopped basil leaves. Pour into a chilled shallow freezer container and freeze for about 2 hours or until mushy.
5   Remove the container from the freezer and beat the mixture with a fork to break down any ice crystals. Return to the freezer and freeze for a

further 4 hours. (If a creamier texture is desired, whisk the egg white until stiff, fold into the beaten mixture and return to the freezer. Freeze as before.)

6   Meanwhile, wash the leeks thoroughly and cut into fine julienne strips of equal length. Cut the carrots and courgettes into julienne strips of the same size.

7   Bring a large pan of water to the boil and add the leeks. Blanch for 1 minute, then remove with a slotted spoon and drain on absorbent kitchen paper. Blanch the carrots in the same water for about 4 minutes, remove and drain well. Similarly, blanch the courgettes for 2 minutes and then drain well.

8   Put the vegetable julienne in a bowl, add the vinaigrette and salt and pepper to taste and toss gently to mix. Cover and chill in the refrigerator until required.

9   To serve, allow the tomato ice to soften in the refrigerator for 30 minutes. Arrange small scoops of tomato ice on chilled individual side plates with a 'nest' of julienne vegetables. Garnish with fresh basil.

MONKFISH THERMIDOR

The sauce for this fish dish is made by the blended method, which eliminates the inclusion of fat. Using strong-flavoured cheeses such as Gruyère and Parmesan means only a little cheese is required.

Serves 6

335 kcals per serving

1.1 kg (2½ lb) monkfish fillet, cubed	450 ml (¾ pint) semi-skimmed milk
3 shallots, skinned and chopped	45 ml (3 tbsp) cornflour
15 ml (1 tbsp) chopped fresh tarragon or 5 ml (1 tsp) dried	10 ml (2 tsp) made English mustard
225 ml (8 fl oz) dry white wine	25 g (1 oz) Parmesan cheese, grated
	75 g (3 oz) Gruyère cheese, grated

1   Put the monkfish in a saucepan with the shallots, tarragon and wine, cover and simmer for 18–20 minutes or until the flesh flakes easily. Using a slotted spoon, remove the fish and reserve the cooking liquid.

2   Blend together the milk and cornflour and add to the cooking liquid with the mustard and Parmesan cheese. Bring to the boil and stir until smooth and thick. Add the fish and transfer to a 1.2 litre (2 pint) shallow ovenproof serving dish.

3   Sprinkle over the Gruyère cheese and cook under a preheated hot grill for 5–10 minutes or until golden brown.

*F*IGS WITH RASPBERRY SAUCE

To reduce the calorie content of this dessert, sweeten it with artificial sweetener, omitting the honey, and use low-fat yogurt instead of Greek yogurt.

Serves 6

90 kcals per serving

12 ripe fresh figs, washed
350 g (12 oz) raspberries, thawed if frozen
90 ml (6 tbsp) Greek yogurt
15 ml (1 tbsp) clear honey
extra raspberries and fresh mint leaves, to decorate

1 Make four cuts in each fig, from the stalk end almost down to the rounded end. Open each fig to resemble a flower and set aside.

2 Purée the raspberries in a blender or food processor until smooth, or rub through a nylon sieve. Pour the purée into a bowl and add the yogurt and honey. Mix well.

3 Arrange the prepared figs on six individual serving plates. Pour a little raspberry sauce on to each plate and decorate with raspberries and mint leaves. Serve the remaining sauce separately.

*C*ALORIE CONTENT TABLE

Item	Average Size		Cals
	oz	g	

ALCOHOLIC DRINKS

Item	Average Size		Cals
Beer (¹/₂ pint)	10 fl oz	280 ml	100
Cider, sweet (¹/₂ pint)	10 fl oz	280 ml	100
Sherry (standard measure)	2 fl oz	50 ml	65
Whisky (standard glass)	1 fl oz	25 ml	65
Wine (standard glass)	5 fl oz	140 ml	100

BISCUITS, CAKES, PASTRY & PIES

Item	Average Size		Cals
Biscuits, digestive, plain (1 biscuit)			70
chocolate (1 biscuit)			130
gingernut (1 biscuit)			65
semi-sweet, eg rich tea (1 biscuit)			50
Cake, sponge	2	60	260
plain fruit	3	90	300
Dundee or similar	4	110	390
currant bun (1)	4	110	340
doughnut with jam (1)	4¹/₂	130	450
Pastry, short, cooked	1	30	150
flaky, cooked	1	30	160
Pie, apple	6	170	300
gooseberry	6	170	300
steak & kidney (individual)	8	230	735
Cornish pasty	6	170	570
Sausage roll (flaky pastry, 1 small)	2	60	270

BREAD

Item	Average Size		Cals
Bread, white (1 med slice)	1	30	70
brown (1 med slice)	1	30	65
wheatgerm (1 med slice)	1	30	65
wholemeal (1 med slice)	1	30	60

CEREALS

Item	Average Size		Cals
Bran-enriched cereal (small bowl)	2	60	160
Cornflakes (small bowl)	1	30	105
Muesli (small bowl)	2	60	210
Porridge, instant (small bowl)	1	30	110
Sugar coated cereals (small bowl)	1	30	100

CHEESE

Item	Average Size		Cals
Austrian, smoked	1	30	75
Camembert	1	30	85
Cheddar	1	30	120
Cottage (small carton)	4	110	100
Cream	1	30	125
Curd (small carton)	4	110	100
Edam	1	30	85
Gouda	1	30	85
Stilton	1	30	130

CREAM

Item	Average Size		Cals
Cream, single	1	30	60
double	1	30	125
clotted	1	30	160

CRISPS & NUTS

Item	Average Size		Cals
Crisps, potato (small pkt)			125
Nuts, chestnuts (shelled)	2	60	100
peanuts (roasted)	1	30	160

EGGS

Item	Average Size		Cals
Egg, boiled or poached, no fat (size 1 or 2)			90
(size 3 or 4)			80
Egg, fried (size 3)			130
Omelette, made using 2 eggs (size 3), no fat			160

Item	Average Size		Cals
	oz	g	

FATS

Item	Average Size		Cals
Butter, salted or unsalted			
(1 pat or 1 tsp)	1/4	10	50
Lard	1	30	255
Margarine (1 pat or 1 tsp)	1/4	10	50
Low-fat spreads			
(1 pat or 1 tsp)	1/4	10	20
Oil, any (2 tbsp)	1	30 ml	255

FISH

Item	Average Size		Cals
Cod, steamed or poached	5	140	130
Crab, canned	4	110	100
Haddock, fresh or smoked, steamed or poached	5	140	145
Herring, grilled	5	140	280
Kipper, grilled	5	140	290
Pilchards, canned in tomato sauce	4	110	140
Prawns, boiled	2	60	60
Salmon, steamed or poached	5	140	280
Sardines, canned in tomato sauce	2	60	100
Trout, grilled or poached (1 small)	10	280	200
Fish fingers, grilled (2)	2	60	100

FRUIT

Item	Average Size		Cals
Apple, raw (1 medium)	6	170	60
stewed, no sugar	5	140	50
Apricot, raw (2 medium)	4	110	20
stewed, no sugar	5	140	35
Banana (1 medium)	6	170	75
Blackberries, stewed, no sugar	4	110	30
Cherries, raw	4	110	45
Fruit salad, canned	4	110	110
Gooseberries, stewed, no sugar	4	110	15
Grapefruit (1/2 medium)	5	140	15
Grapes	4	110	70
Lemon (1 medium)	3	90	15
Melon, honeydew (1 medium slice, weighed with skin	5	140	25
Orange (1 large)	8	230	40
Peach, raw (1 large)	4	110	35
Pear (1 medium)	4	110	45

Item	Average Size		Cals
	oz	g	
Pineapple, raw (1 slice)	4	110	55
Raspberries, raw	4	110	25
Rhubarb, stewed, no sugar	5	140	10
Strawberries	6	170	45

FRUIT, DRIED

Item	Average Size		Cals
Dates, dried (weighed with stones)	2	60	120
Figs, dried (weighed with stones)	2	60	120
Peaches (dried), stewed, no sugar	4	110	90
Prunes, stewed, no sugar	4	110	95
Raisins, sultanas, currants	1	30	70

GREEN & SALAD VEGETABLES

Item	Average Size		Cals
Beans, runner, boiled	4	110	20
Brussels sprouts, boiled	4	110	20
Cabbage, boiled	4	110	15
Cauliflower, boiled	4	110	10
Celery, raw	2	60	5
Cucumber, raw	1	30	3
Lettuce, raw	4	110	10
Mushrooms, raw	2	60	8
Onions, raw	1	30	5
Peas, fresh, boiled	3	90	45
frozen, boiled	3	90	45
Peppers, raw	2	60	10
Spring greens, boiled	4	110	40
Tomatoes (1 large)	2	60	8

LOW-CALORIE DRINKS

Item	Average Size		Cals
Bovril, cup made with 1 tsp			5
Coffee, no milk, no sugar			neg
Low-calorie mixers			neg
Orange juice	5 fl oz	140 ml	50
Oxo, cup made with 1 cube			15
Tea, no milk, no sugar			neg
Tomato juice	5 fl oz	140 ml	20
Water			0

MEAT

Item	Average Size		Cals
Bacon, lean gammon, grilled	4	110	260

Item	Average Size		Cals
	oz	g	

Item	Average Size		Cals
	oz	g	

Item	oz	g	Cals
streaky, grilled (2 rashers)	3	90	130
Beef, average joint, roasted	4	110	400
minced, cooked	4	110	260
steak, grilled	6	170	330
stewing steak	4	110	260
Lamb, leg, roasted	4	110	325
chop, grilled (weighed without bone)	4	110	400
Pork, average joint, roasted	4	110	450
chop, grilled (weighed without bone)	6	170	565
Veal, fillet, roasted	4	110	260
cutlet, fried in breadcrumbs	6	170	365
Beefburger, average, grilled	4	110	290
Sausage, pork, grilled (2 average)	4	110	360
Ham, lean	4	110	300
Corned beef	4	110	240

MILK

Item	oz	g	Cals
Milk, whole, silver top	½pt	280 ml	190
Milk, semi-skimmed	½pt	280 ml	132
Milk, skimmed	½pt	280 ml	100

POULTRY, GAME & OFFAL

Item	oz	g	Cals
Chicken, roast	5	140	210
Duck, roast	5	140	270
Heart, ox (stewed)	6	170	300
Liver, lamb's (fried)	4	110	260
Kidney, lamb's (fried)	4	110	180
Rabbit, stewed	6	170	300
Turkey, roast	4	110	160

RICE & PASTA

Item	oz	g	Cals
Pasta, white, boiled	6	170	200
brown, boiled	6	170	200
Rice, white, boiled	4	110	140
brown, boiled	4	110	140

ROOT VEGETABLES & PULSES

Item	oz	g	Cals
Beans, baked, cooked (small tin)	5	140	100
butter, cooked	4	110	100
red kidney, cooked	4	110	100
Carrots, boiled	4	110	20
Leeks, boiled	4	110	30
Lentils, split, boiled	4	110	120
Onions, boiled	4	110	15
Parsnips, boiled	4	110	60
Potatoes, boiled	4	110	100
roast	4	110	180
Sweet corn, canned	4	110	80

SOUPS

Item	oz	g	Cals
Chicken, cream (tinned, average bowl)	10 fl oz	280 ml	140
Consommé (tinned, average bowl)	10 fl oz	280 ml	70
Lentil (packet, average bowl)	10 fl oz	280 ml	300
Minestrone (packet, average bowl)	10 fl oz	280 ml	65
Oxtail (packet, average bowl)	10 fl oz	280 ml	150

SUGAR, SWEETS, CHOCOLATE & PRESERVES

Item	oz	g	Cals
Sugar, white or brown (1 tsp)	¼	10	20
Chocolate	1	30	150
Toffees (assorted)	1	30	120
Sweets, boiled	1	30	95
Jam or marmalade (1 tbsp)			20
Honey	1	30	80
Syrup	1	30	85

INDEX